Praise for
Anne & Ivan Kronenfeld

"**This is an enthralling account**, not just of an extraordinary woman, but of a tumultuous era." —Howard Kissel, columnist, *New York Daily News*

"**An astounding story crammed with intrigue,** human triumph, and delicious historical detail." —Stephen J. Dubner, author of *Turbulent Souls: A Catholic Son's Return to His Jewish Family*

"**A beautifully written book about a fascinating woman** who would not be deprived her gift... courageous in secret and triumphant in life. A remarkable human being." —Richard Mulligan, Star of *Soap* and *Empty Nest*

"**A stunning success of a book** about an indomitable spirit .... It makes you think ...." Paul Price, script writer for *Empty Nest*

"**A powerfully written novel.**" —Terry L. White, author of *Ancient Memories* and *No More Dishes to Wash.*

"**Sweeping in scope,** this fictionalized account will leave you wanting more." —Arline Chase, author of *Spirit of Fire* and *Ghost Dancer.*

"**This book opened wonderful doors to me on the role of an outstanding woman** in the field of medicine, especially in her time." — Marjorie Doughty, author of *Reenactment.*

"**...outstanding...**" —Robert Legleitner, author of *The Kydon Chronicles.*

The Secret Life of Dr. James Miranda Barry

Anne and Ivan Kronenfeld

ebooksonthe.net
an imprint of
Write Words, Inc.
Cambridge, MD

Third Paper Edition, August, 2004

Publishers Note: This book is a work of fiction based entirely on the author's imagination. Any resemblance to actual persons is purely coincidental. Real places mentioned in the book are depicted fictionally and are not intended to portray actual times or places.

ebooksonthe.net is a subsidiary of:

Write Words, Inc.
2934 Old Route 50
Cambridge, MD 21613

ISBN 1-59431-090-4

Fax : 410-221-7510

"A good surgeon requires an eagle's eye,
a lion's heart, and a lady's hand."
—Proverb

Manchester Guardian
August 21, 1865

"A Strange Story—an incident is just now being discussed in British military circles, so extraordinary that were not the truth capable of being vouched for by official authority, the narration would certainly be deemed absolutely incredible. Our officers quartered at the Cape may remember a certain Dr. James Barry. He enjoyed a reputation for considerable skill in his profession, especially for firmness and rapid directions.

The gentleman in question pursued a legitimate medical education at one of our most prestigious universities and received its diploma. Passed through the grades of assistant surgeon and surgeon in various regiments quartered all over the globe and had acquired celebrity for skill as a surgical operator, ultimately achieving the rank of Inspector General of Hospitals, in his last post, the Dominion of Canada.

After retirement he settled in London, where in the month past he perished in the dysentery epidemic and upon his death was discovered to be a woman. The motive that occasioned and the time when commenced this singular deception, are both shrouded in mystery.

But thus it stands as an indubitable fact, that a woman was for forty years an officer in the British service."

CHAPTER ONE

"Pray, forgive me, Doctor," rumbled Surgeon Major Nigel, looking down at Pandora whose diminutive size stood in startling contrast to the man's grand height and prodigious dimensions. He was well over six feet, but it was not his height alone which made such an impressive presentation. Everything about him was king-sized: his hands, his feet, even the mustache which dominated his rough-hewn face was oversized. "But I do find it quizzical that a fellow such as you would be wanting to join the Army Medical Corps."

"I'm not quite clear," Pandora said, "what you mean when you refer to me as 'a fellow such as you'?"

"Why, I only meant, Doctor, that we seldom see people with constitutions, how can I say, as delicate as yours. But, that aside, it seems to me a man with your qualifications is surely confronted with infinitely more comfortable possibilities than those that would be provided by an army career."

"Tropical diseases, sir," Pandora retorted.

"Now I am the one who is confused," said the surgeon major, leaning on his desk, his powerful hands crossed in front of him.

"My rationale is really quite simple, sir. We English are conducting our affairs with increasing regularity in equatorial regions. This presents our men with quite a different circumstance from that to which the British body is accustomed. The diseases peculiar to these climates present to any physician a unique challenge to probe the unknown and unstudied."

"Well said, young man, and all to the common good. But you yourself must be aware that you present a figure incompatible with what is considered the standard military stock."

"Ah, Doctor," Pandora said, "an understandable observation. But if you will calculate my worth based on my credentials..."

"What is needed on the field of battle, young man, cannot be found in paper qualifications. Character, the kind born in a man's bones and gristle, is what is required in the officers of the Army Medical Corps. It seems to me," his fingers drummed on the painted miniature of three women whom Pandora assumed to be his wife and daughters, "that you, with your impressive background, could easily have a flourishing practice right here in London, comfortably catering to the hysterical maladies of the rich. Now wouldn't that be more suitable for someone like yourself than heading out like Saint Francis of Assisi to some remote corner of the globe?"

"I'll grant you that your conclusions are quite logical, Surgeon Major, sir, but I am afraid that I would find the practice you most aptly describe both tedious and boring. I realize full well that my physical presentation is not what one usually encounters in a military mode, but an individual's spirit cannot be so readily seen. A man can be large of bulk and sparse of soul. I wish to prove of what stuff I am made."

Dr. Nigel raised his eyebrows and began examining the young doctor's papers. In the pause, Pandora looked around the stark room. Just behind the surgeon major, set incongruously atop his instrument case, were six splendidly carved wooden soldiers, each one dressed in appropriate military attire. One was a British Grenadier, another an Irish soldier of James II, another a Scots Fencible in full plaid kilt, a Moor, a Roman with shield, and, lastly, a Gurkha with a wide-bladed kukri sword.

"Your vitae is impressive indeed, Dr. Barry," the major said. "Pupil dresser to Sir Astley Cooper. Perhaps I have been making some precipitant assumptions. Why don't we proceed to the scale and we'll begin the examination. As a matter of fact, I am an Edinburgh man myself," he said with a friendly wink.

Pandora latched onto this commonalty and began to formulate a plan. She could see the tide was turning in her favor; the dolls, Edinburgh, she had it.

"Just seven stone you are," he said, making a notation. Pandora heard disappointment in his voice. "Step to the wall sir, let's have a measure. Just under the five foot mark. Well now, son," the major sat on the corner of his examining table, one leg dangling, "I must say with candor I have rather grave doubts whether someone of your scant proportion could withstand the rigors of foreign service. Particularly in the tropics..."

"Sir!" she cried, before he could continue. "These dolls are exquisite! I cannot take my eyes off them!"

"Oh, my collection," he said, looking up at them proudly like a father does his brood. "Well, thank you, thank you. It's just a small hobby I enjoy during my leisure."

"You mean, sir, these sublime figures were done by your own hand?"

"Well, yes, but it's not all that inspiring," Dr. Nigel said, a wave of embarrassment streaking his face.

"Sir!" Pandora said, "you are much too modest. Why, craft of such a caliber demands high approbation."

"I feel that you are a flatterer, sir. You are much too kind."

"May I be so bold as to request holding one," Pandora asked.

"With pleasure," he agreed, taking one enormous step to the cabinet and exposing his massive back to Pandora as he retrieved a doll. "This is the one of which I am most proud." He handed it to her caringly. "An Indian Gurkha, one of the world's finest fighting men. This is the famous kukri." He pointed to the delicately carved weapon.

"Magnificent!" Pandora exclaimed, taking the figure and standing it upright on the examining table. "May I say, Dr. Nigel, if your skill with a scalpel is matched by your ability with a carving knife, then I am sure I am in the presence of one of England's finest military surgeons."

"Well, young man, I wouldn't be so bold as to declare such a statement. But I will admit to the pupil dresser of such a renowned surgeon as Sir Astely Cooper that it has been said, 'If you need to lose a limb, Old Doc Nigel is the one to have do it.'"

"Dr. Nigel, did you perchance ever perform in the 'Dead House' at Edinburgh, a cesarean section?"

"Lord not, Sir!" Dr. Nigel exploded, "That's a procedure I wouldn't even perform on the deceased. Why, to think of tearing out from the womb a babe that God is withholding is pagan and barbaric. I'll have no part of it!"

"Aren't you forgetting the proverb," Pandora asked, picking up his Gurkha, "'*Quem non dim pervasti postvesti illium occedesti*': To neglect to save a person when it is in your power to do so, is to be an accessory to death. Major, we are speaking here of the only operation where two lives may be saved." Pandora moved with dispatch and grabbed a pillow off the examining table.

"Dr. Barry, I know of no one who has succeeded with this cruel procedure."

"That is only because we have all been cowards, standing around, wringing our hands like old women, instead of performing our duty as surgeons. Let me show you exactly what I mean." A whirlwind of efficiency, she took his carving knife from his desk, slit open the top of a pillow, and gently stuffed the Gurkha into the feathers. Then quickly she slid that inside an empty pillowcase.

"This is not a dilemma of technique, but a crisis of courage and indecision." She swung herself onto the table and lay down in the labor position, placing the Gurkha-impregnated pillow on her belly. "Doctor, bring your scalpel."

Mystified and intrigued by the goings on, the Surgeon Major secured one from his case. "Now," she instructed, "make a longitudinal incision on the outside of the rectus muscles."

She saw him look a bit stunned at the large feather-filled obtrusion. "Between the navel and the angle of the osillium," she encouraged. He bent forward and executed her instructions on the first layer.

"Now, sir," she hardly gave him time to breathe, "divide the membrane adipose, about eight or nine fingers in length. There you would pass through the oblique and transverse muscles. Carefully," she warned from raised elbows, looking down on his work. "Now through the peritoneum, a small puncture must be made." He did just so into the pillow, at which point several goose feathers escaped.

"Excellent, Doctor! Further divide until the opening appears large enough to extract the fetus." Dr. Nigel, now fully engrossed, gently felt through the feathers, which began to fly every which way, until he found the doll. At this point, he victoriously pulled it from the pillow and with genteel dispatch presented it to Dr. Barry. "Well done, sir," said the patient. "Now would you suture, please?" Both doctors broke into a broad laugh.

"Well, blood and wounds!" Dr. Nigel said, feathers vibrating on his dampened mustache. "It does seem quite a simple matter."

"It is indeed, but only if done with such care and dispatch as yours."

"Thank you, doctor."

"Well, Major," Pandora stood at a modified attention, "do you think the British Army could find use for someone the likes of me after all?"

"I must admit," the surgeon major said, "you are a most remarkable young man."

CHAPTER TWO

The year 1794 had been a bad year for bread, wine and children. The soil of France nourished best chaos and blood, and all her citizens lived in fear of the great blade that instantly separated brother from sister, husband from wife, and mother from child.

The quiet river drew witness as it wound its way westward, bisecting Paris right from left. It swallowed the severed body parts of those tossed into it like unwanted rubbish. It cleansed itself of their blood with its current and in its twisting path to the sea it carried away their agonizing cries.

Under a bridge in a gentle bend of the river between the Jardins des Tuileries and the Champs de Mars lived a child alone and abandoned. It was dark and dank under the bridges that passed over the Seine. Even the sun was unwilling to share its warmth with the creatures who dwelt beneath. Fierce, red-eyed rats watched keenly in the darkness as little hands dropped bits of scavenged food into makeshift fires, which laced the humid air with heavy acrid smoke. Flying insects and giant cockroaches scurried from the light to darker, safer sanctuaries. And the passing Seine licked at the walls of the quay as if it hungered for the human waste deposited along its edges. It ignored the nocturnal screams of the abandoned children who huddled for safety under the bridges, only to be tormented in their sleep by the savage pictures of torture and dismemberment they witnessed by day.

From under one of these bridges a small red-headed urchin appeared in the hazy morning light. Stretching and shaking herself, catlike, she made her way to the edge of the quay and captured in her palms a trickle of water from a nearby drainpipe.

Bringing it to her lips, she paused briefly to savor the wetness in her parched mouth. Then she examined the new patches of molted insect bites she'd acquired during the night.

***

Paris was filled with such orphans as this, casualties of changes they could not possibly fathom. They were not concerned with the affairs of state, the philosophies of Rousseau, or the deep issues that embraced the bitter imbroglio between Girondists and Jacobins. These were things far beyond the realm of their comprehension. They were children whose singular concern was survival in a place that had no time to care for them. Many mustered their collective strength into packs. Like dogs they scavenged for scraps of food, biting and scrapping with each other for the largest piece. Then they huddled next to one another at night against the cold and their fear of darkness. The youngest, those who had not even the recollection of a mother's kiss, always worked their way into the very center of these sleeping entanglements, where for at least the time being, they found warmth in the touch of their comrades.

This girl was different. She was, like so many of the others, an orphan of the Terror, deprived of name and hearth; but, unlike her confreres, she belonged to no band, was a member of no pack. She depended on herself. She hunted alone. Since those bloody September days in the year of 1792, she had survived by her curious birthright, an independent nature coupled with a quick mind. The breaking dawn burst across the edge of the river with uncommon perfection for this June day.

The sun, cresting the horizon, cast its golden light across the cheeks of the child as she leaned forward again to satiate her thirst. Her penetrating hazel eyes darted rapidly about, taking in the surroundings. She listened to the growing clang of the tocsin bells that were calling all the citizens of Paris this morning. She was hungry and she knew clanging bells meant an assembly.

Soon she heard the tramp of masses of feet coming toward the bridge, and as they came into view above her, she stepped into the shadows to conceal herself and plan her strategy. Men and women appeared, adorned with scarves and sashes of the tricolor red, white and blue. Children, some clinging to their mothers' skirts, were dressed in pure white, shockingly bright in the intensifying sunlight. The girls had wreaths in their hair, many of the boys and all of the men had picks, and everyone held a bouquet of violets, roses and corn.

The urchin watched from her hiding place as the marchers began to cross the bridge, and she began to surmise where she might take advantage of the situation. Soon a great float pulled by eight cows came into view. Its four tiers were draped with tricolored banners, each overlain with every type of farm implement. On the upper tier, high above the crowd and flanked by two cornucopias overflowing with fruits and vegetables, was a large statue of Liberty clothed in provocative gauze. In her outstretched hand she held a clod of French soil and behind her was a live tree growing from the center of the float. Accompanying the spectacle was a compact group of young maidens with myrtle head wreaths and elderly women holding garlands of leafy vines. They were encircled with red, white and blue ribbons carried by children who themselves were ornamented with violets.

Following the float came a cart of blind children being pulled by a group of citizens. The children had been groomed and dressed in fresh clothing and along with their bouquets they carried a piece of bread. A great stir of sympathy was being showered upon these children who normally felt the heel of a boot as they tried to beg for their survival.

What fools these adults can be, the child thought, amused at the overly solicitous women fussing about the cart. Large dumb creatures is all they are, she mused, her busy eyes taking in the whole scene.

Then another thought occurred to her: "Today blindness means breakfast." And as she scurried up the embankment she began to master the necessary transformation. Spurning beggars arriving in unison with the cart upon the bridge, she pulled herself onto the already overburdened conveyance, closed her eyes almost shut and tilted her head back. Feeling her way forward, she purposely stepped on the toes of a smartly dressed attendant in a blue jacket and Jacobin cap. As he turned, she said in a shrill and demanding tone, "Bread, bread, am I not blind, too?" The attendant picked up her hand, pressed a crusty bread into it, kissed her forcefully on the forehead, then patted her filthy little head. The cart lurched as cannon fire signaled the official commencement of the festivities and the child took secure hold of her benefactor's hand. The grand procession lumbered along as section joined section from either side of the Seine. The labor of pulling the immense floats into line caused long delay for the masses of Parisians all heading toward the Jardins des Tuileries oratory of Robespierre, but the day had been blessed with mild temperatures as if the new Supreme Being Himself approved of this feast in His honor.

Along the periphery the crowd threw coins at each passing float. Throughout the mob, singing could be heard and sporadically small groups burst into the revolutionary dance, the charmagnole.

Past the throngs, the floats, the gathering soloists, and choristers of the National Institute of Music (who would later sing at the Champs de Mars, upon the sides of an enormous mountain constructed as a symbol of the majority of the Convention), past the sections led by specially selected members of the Jacobin Society, past 100 drummers, a detachment of cavaliers, firemen and cannoneers, lay the first destination—the Tuileries Gardens. A huge scaffolding had been erected in front of the central pavilion, in the form of two staircases with circular ramps between them. It rose from the ground to the third level of the pavilion.

Groups of choristers and 200 musicians were already arranged on the first floor platform. Above them, seated behind the empty chair of the President, were the eleven representatives of the Convention. It took until noon for all to gather. The Tailors could not contain them, and they overflowed into the Rue de la Reine, climbing trees, trying to secure a vantage point from which to see Robespierre.

Finally, from the Grand Salon of the Pavilion, wearing a nattily tailored blue coat, a tricolored sash, with three large matching plumes positioned in his hat, appeared Maximilien Robespierre. His familiar green glasses covered his eyes, and he held a bouquet of bluets and corn poppies in his hand. He stood above the crowd, and all heads turned upward in greeting. Looking down on this human sea, Robespierre smiled as if he felt an uncharacteristic sense of elation, and when he began to speak, his voice trembled with overwhelming enthusiasm.

"The universe is here assembled!" he began in his thick provincial accent.

"Oh, nature, how beautiful and sublime is thy power." In priest-like blessing, he held aloft the small bouquet. "Tyrants, do you not tremble at the thought of this festival? French republicans, at last this ever blessed and happy day has arrived, the day which we, the French People, consecrate to the Supreme Being." His short frame was shaking now with nervous agitation. "Never has the world, which He created, presented an aspect so worthy of His greatness."

"Countrymen! Today let us surrender ourselves under the protection of God to transports of the purest delights; tomorrow we shall again combat vice and tyranny; we shall show the world the republican virtues, and this will be still more to His honor!"

Behind Robespierre there was a flare of light as one of those assembled on the scaffolding handed him a torch. Striding forward, he ignited a pasteboard statue called Atheism. As it burned, a mechanical device cranked up through the midst of its flames, the incombustible figure of Wisdom. Still holding the torch in one hand, bouquet in the other, Robespierre acknowledged the ovation of the legions by commencing with another appeal.

"Let us be generous to the good, kind towards the unfortunate, inexorable towards the wicked and just to the whole world!" Although Robespierre's small stature was diminished even further by the height of the scaffolding, his presence had overwhelmed everything and, for what appeared to be a perfectly orchestrated moment, the citizens of Paris began to sing.

Come down to us, oh, Liberty,
Come down, great nature's child,
Lo! France has won her power,
Immortal, undefiled
The awful ruins lie around
With ancient error scored,
Thy altar is restored.

Through all these goings on the little girl alone gave no attention to the demigod's speech. She was on her hands and knees crawling around the bottom of the cart packing her cheeks with bread and her pockets with coins. When her bounty was satisfied, she sat on her haunches and watched her blue-coated benefactor scream himself hoarse with the rest of the throng. At the height of his elation, his attention far from his charges, she pushed herself between a cluster of legs off the back of the cart where she quickly merged into the crowd and headed off to attend to her other business.

CHAPTER THREE

All through history, particularly at times of great stress and upheaval, there has existed a consistent peculiarity, an unwritten code that the mad, the very old and the very young are looked upon as outside the main body of the mass. Thus, unencumbered by ordinary social constraints, they remain disconnected and oft times unseen, left to survive by their own means and wit. Such a covenant served well for this small red-headed urchin. Indeed, as she was an unusually percipient child, she observed this mystery and saw it as the cornerstone of her survival. Taking full advantage of her place among the excluded in this time of change, she created a world suitable for her existence.

Leaving the crowd behind, she quick-stepped her way down the deserted quay. Finding a dark niche behind a stack of molasses barrels, she sat down and made neat piles of the sous between her stretched legs. Never before had she held so much wealth. It intoxicated her. She drooled at the thought of all that food: white bread, cream puff pastries, hot soups, perhaps a new dress. Weeks and weeks worth of money sat there looking back at her.

"Oh what a lucky day this is, the luckiest that has ever been. But where should I keep my treasure? Should I hide it? Or should I take it with me?" She decided to take it with her; it was safer. She carefully placed each pile on a rag, and tied it into a tight bundle. As the day would soon turn to dusk she feared she would be late to the cemetery, and the gates would be closed, preventing her harvest of newly laid bouquets, thus leaving her with no flowers to sell on her evening rounds of bars and theaters. But she reassured herself by hefting the bundle of coins and placed it deep in the pocket of her oversized smock. "Even if there might be no flower business tonight, today will have been a golden one nonetheless."

Rising, she giggled with pride at the cleverness of the morning's performance and rewarded herself by popping another piece of bread into her mouth. Then she took up a leisurely pace, allowing herself to enjoy its taste.

Although there had been a momentary respite from the violence, so many had already fallen that all the cemeteries were filled and those unlucky ones who had no relatives to receive their remains were thrown into common graves. Such had been the fate of her mother, of whom she had no memory or recollection. This served as a mixed blessing. While it left her with no knowledge of her family, it also absolved her of the torment connected with them. She did not weep for them as did those whom she now watched intently, while they placed their small floral tokens on the mounds.

Standing close to a broken moss-covered headstone, she remained a respectful distance from the last two mourners in wait of their departure. One, a stoop-figured fellow, leaning on his gnarled walking stick, looked over his shoulder before quickly making the forbidden sign of the cross under the intimate protection of his cloak. The other, a black bonneted woman accompanied by her small child, knelt in the fading daylight and kissed the still earth while the toddler, oblivious to all, explored the nearby grass with both hands. With grievous sobs, the woman snatched up her child, pulling dirt and grass from his clenched fist. Then enfolding him in her shawl and pressing his silky blond head to her shoulder, she hurried out of the gate, her vanishing silhouette weighted down from the mantle of death.

Now that the coast was clear the urchin crossed the sacred ground, gathering as many fresh bouquets as she could. Laying them on the ground she divided them by group—daisies the largest, violets the second, and a few beaten roses. She did not worry much about the gatekeepers for on one of her first visits here some time ago when they had caught her, she had won them over by performing, with appropriate passion, an impromptu sad tale. She told them of how she'd watched each member of her family being led to the guillotine, grandfather first, then her father, and finally her dear mother and that the sale of these flowers was her only means of sustenance. It was a startling and touching performance, affecting those hardened keepers profoundly as they had looked down on her, a small, thin child with strands of red curls sticking to her tear-streaked face. But they'd warned her sternly to make sure she waited until all the grievers were gone before beginning her collections. She'd acquiesced with her most respectful and angelic face. In fact she had won them over so completely that not only did she come and go unmolested, but on occasion, particularly if they were thick with drink, the keepers could be counted on for a small favor, a morsel of food or a glass of wine. Flower selling was a good business, but not without risk. She had noticed that when the weather was poor, mourners did not come to pay their respects. And so she had learned to save the more hearty stems for those unpredictable contingencies.

Thanks to the continued mild weather and the festive mood left over from the day-long feast, all the restaurants were crammed with patrons. The child pushed in and out of her usual haunts, selling her flowers to regulars and ordinary passersby with goodly dispatch. She spotted one of her favorite dandies, a tall, slim, dark mustached fellow named Gerard, escorting an exquisitely gowned woman with sparkling things in her upswept hair.

"Monsieur Gerard, Monsieur Gerard!" she called him, dashing across the street, dodging carts, feet and the muck with masterly aplomb.

"Monsieur, for your beautiful lady," she said, holding the last perky bunch of violets up to him.

"Ah, ma petite, just whom I've been looking for on such an opportune night." He patted her, as usual, atop her disarray of red curls and slipped a large coin into her waiting palm.

"Merci!" She curtseyed charmingly, then headed with her last dozen fading daisies and three brown-edged pink roses to the Pigeon Breast.

"Vin," she called up to the barkeep who leaned over the bar with his sweaty face beaming down at her.

"Here, la petite."

He handed her the red drink, which she downed with dispatch. Then she stuck one daisy in his ear and turned to head home. The whole of today was definitely a success. But growing fatigue and the wine had made her forget always to think practically. She remembered that she'd promised never to indulge her feelings where matters of money were concerned.

"Never let inclination rise above obligation," she reminded herself, shaking out the droopy daisies and stopping just short of the exit. She about-faced and scanned the barroom. There were the customary whores draped over chair backs or leaning in little clusters of seats arranged haphazardly along the narrow room. Nearly all were engaged in their routine preliminary to sales. Since whores seldom buy flowers, the child's prospects for her few remaining buds looked grim. Then she spotted a sympathetic-faced bargeman at the end of the bar drinking freely with one hand and strumming the bar with the other.

"My father was a sailor," she said approaching him. "Died in a shipwreck on the South China Sea. Had tattoos just like you, mister. You want to hear me sing a sea chantey?"

The well-tanned lad grinned glassy-eyed at her. She was correct. His smile was benevolent and he hoisted her up on the bar.

> "Oh, when I'm far away at sea,
> My sweet Abigail,
> I know She waits for me,"

Her voice, though sweet enough was bereft of accurate pitch, and because her confidence was such that she sang loudly, her errors in tone drew everyone's attention and the whores laughed delightedly.

> "Her lips are moist and red,
> her heart is swelled with love,
> and I know as sure as the sky's above
> there's no one in her bed."

"Bravo!" the room called, the child bowed, and the river man snapped up some coins and flipped them one by one into her hands. Then he kissed her cheek and deposited her back to the ground. As she was leaving the child saw him passing out the daisies to all the "ladies" with a great swell of romantic largesse.

Patting her lump of money she headed "home" to her place of rest under the Pont Neuf. She took the last of her bread and began a final snack.

"How didja do? Whatcha got, carrot-head?" a flat-faced boy said, jumping in her path from the shadows of the alley, stopping her cold with the slap of a flat board across her chest. Her mouth went dry. She knew there was never just one of these. Sure enough, she saw two, three—seven emerge all around her. "Trapped!" she cursed to herself.

"Oh it's been a bad day," she said with forced confidence, trying to chart a flight. "Just a few sous, a couple a crusts." She held out her half gnawed bread.

"Oh, yeah!" The boy slapped the piece onto the ground, his stick stinging her fingers.

"Let's just see what kind of liar you are! Hoist her up, me boys!" The others moved in and swooped her upside down in one quick motion, then shook her hard, banging her head on the cobbles. She heard the coins hitting, one by one, then felt the precious tied rag slip from its hiding place and land with a solid thud at the leader's feet.

"Oh ho!" he cried, slashing it open with his knife, releasing a rain of coin.

"And what could you possibly have done for this fine money!" The boys laughed at the dirty thought.

"Gimme that now, it's mine!" She reached for some of the coins, but the leader caught her with a crack, the edge of the board opening her forehead.

"It's mine. I want it now!" she cried.

"Oh, you want it? Paul!" the boy called. "She wants it."

She felt a hard kick on her rump and her knees collapsed; she flew forward, head first into the wet, refuse-clogged canal, which ran down the middle of the street. Quickly returning to her feet, front soaked with foulness, she stood bleeding and listened to the laughing boys as they counted her money from down one of the odious black alleys.

"Motherless pigs, you miserable, tailless rats!" she screamed as she sank to her knees and started to cry in earnest. Frantically, she began to feel about in the filthy muck of the canal in hopes of reclaiming some of her lost wages. After a long search that yielded three sous, she gave up and headed for the Pont Neuf.

CHAPTER FOUR

A steady rhythm of rain drops landing on her blood-caked and swollen forehead roused her. At first she'd thought it was a dream. She was being punished, she knew not why, by a faceless man, tap-tapping harder and harder with a small silver-thimbled finger on a spot at the hairline above her right eye. She sat up from the pain of the damnable luck the night before. Then she realized it was morning, she was home under the Pont Neuf. It was raining heavily, coming down all around her, through the cracks in the bridge, but she was almost carefree with relief, for even beatings were less fearsome to her than nightmares. They were her nemesis, and she feared them worse than all the real perils she confronted in her hard-fought existence. As she pulled herself out from under the leaks, she watched the rain wash the quay clean, or at least try, and she was glad to see the old bucket at the drain pipe was getting, if not completely clean water, at least fresh. Today would not be a day for the cemetery, so, doing her best to wash up her wound, she set out with her well-stashed three sous, for the baker on the corner, staying close to the embankment on the street side of the quay in order to avoid a complete soaking. She scurried along, darting up steps and was relieved to see the line was short as yet.

"One sou's worth."

She planted the wet coin on the stone counter with authority and held her hand open for the half coarse loaf the indifferent baker planted in it, then, biting off a piece of the end, she put the other into her skirt's inside pocket and headed out to brave the elements and pay her calls to the prisoners.

She had figured out that diversity was in her best interest and found the prisons of Paris a place of opportunity, especially the prison of La Force, because it housed a prestigious group who tipped well.

Haly and Mathilde, the keepers of the key, knew her well, for she had become a reliable asset to them, as they were in constant need of trustworthy little legs to secure messages here and there and perform other errands. Haly was endowed with a turbulent nature, which had undoubtedly suited him well in his former occupation as a manager of a menagerie of African animals. But the child had learned to gauge his moods accurately. She could tell by the color of his eyes when he was raw with drink and responded by keeping a good distance. Each day without fail her first priority was a stop at the prison of La Force.

Once having passed the guards at the gate, she went left and proceeded down the hall with a slow and methodical walk so she could be sure that Ravage, the huge black mongrel who lay by the door of the superintendent's apartment, would know it was her. His head popped up as the child approached; a deep growl, a show of teeth, then, upon recognition, the mangy cur commenced a display of tail wagging and circular dancing. He was an enormous creature, oddly appreciative toward his little friend, which stood in sharp contrast to his usual unfriendly demeanor. Upon entering the apartment, she found Haly and the gendarme Phillipe engaged in a game of piquet. Phillipe, a man of enormous bulk came daily to La Force to deliver new "batches" of prisoners. He snapped a deuce onto the table.

"Aha! I've got you now. I told you today I'd treat you like a stepchild. I shot the moon; now you must pay double." Sweat poured from his enormous face and clung to his walrus mustache, which he twisted at regular intervals. It was in fact the only part of him at all kempt. Today the stakes were high; the new "batches" had brought quite an array of treasure, which Phillipe mockingly displayed. Adorning himself with rings on every finger and necklaces resting on his bilious chest, he even managed to hang long earrings over his ears. Several green bottles stood empty, reflecting the bleak candlelight, which even the occasional crystal sparkle of the cache of jewels couldn't enliven. Haly's face was close to

Phillipe; the powdered wig he wore hung limply under his red Jacobin hat. He liked the feeling of hair, for he had long since forgotten it, and a gentleman's fine wig pleased him.

"I think you cheat, my friend. My luck cannot be so poor. You have won nearly all my earnings of today and what remains has little value." Phillipe's bellow startled the baubles around his neck. Ravage, aroused by the commotion, rose to his feet and started barking fiercely. "Get to work, you lazy swine!" Mathilde, Phillipe's burly wife, howled, the flab shaking from her underarm as she hurled a wet wad of underwear at Phillipe, knocking him off balance and out of his chair.

"Why is it I have no time for cards or drink? The child wishes to go inside. What do you two louts say? At least have her take that yowling beast before I beat it to death." Haly waved absently at the three of them. He was too busy enjoying the sight of his friend Phillipe, sprawled on the floor. In a flash the child, followed by Ravage, made her way inside. She knew only too well a moment's hesitation could keep her from entry and the errands at hand. The gaolers sleepily opened the inner gate, allowing the two unlikely figures through. It took a bit of adjustment for her eyes to accustom themselves to the dark hallway, but she always closed them just before she reached the outside gate. So when she passed from the light into the darkness her eyes had already begun to adjust.

The main room was lit by several candle stumps, which, when agitated by the drafts, moved the shadows on the walls, creating the illusion that there were more prisoners within than actually existed. The inhabitants of this dreary dungeon often remarked to each other about this phenomenon and half seriously agreed that these phantom shadows were the ghosts of former inmates returning to the scene for the dual purpose of comforting their comrades and serving notice on their tormentors.

Achille de Chatelet lay on the straw mattress he had occupied for so long now. The wound festering in his calf and poisoning his blood carried him in and out of delirium. The young girl had brought him some salve, sent by his wife, in a feeble effort to keep him alive yet another day, always harboring the hope that the Terror would end and the prison doors would fly open.

Verginaud had stopped his writings and was listening intently, along with Valeze, to a man she had not seen before. He spoke like no one she had ever heard, his words rolling lyrically off his tongue. He was of a large construction, standing five feet and ten inches high, well proportioned, with massive shoulders and a strong square chest. His complexion, dark and florid, when juxtaposed to the sallow faces around him, shone like a beacon of light.

Though this child had lived a scant seven years, she was not a stranger to death. She was as accustomed to it as other people were to their mundane routines. Each day she saw the unlucky taken in carts to the guillotine. Some collared around the neck railed for justice, some prayed, some were already dead in their manner, but most begged for life.

She shifted the burlap bag hanging from her shoulder around to her front and prepared to distribute the various messages and items within. This large room, though far from one of comfort, was considered a special section, housing the more "important" prisoners; therefore it lacked the grim and bleak dungeon atmosphere of some other parts of La Force. There were black iron wall sconces scattered irregularly with wicks inserted in them, providing a fair amount of light. Each prisoner also had his own candle and holder along with some sort of a seat, be it a stool or the remnant of a discarded chair. A straw pallet was provided for sleeping and there were two medium sized wooden tables in the center where eating or writing was facilitated. Books, papers and pens were permitted, and the resupply of these was a major part of the little girl's enterprise.

She was popular among most of the inmates; her plucky attitude, seasoned with her tough street ways, had charmed them quite easily. But others demonstrated a cool distance, sprinkled by a measure of disdain toward her, because she was a nameless street urchin entitled only to derision from her betters.

The child wasted no time addressing her chores. She delivered two books to a gentleman nearest the door. Barely acknowledging her, he dropped a gratuity in the little pouch hanging around her waist. She had noticed this fellow growing more and more withdrawn in the last few weeks. She acquiesced to his mood and did not attempt to humor or disturb him. Experience had taught her to go about her business with detached efficiency. Her next delivery was a message. Most of these were written notes from loved ones who quickly scrawled a sentiment or cri du coeur to their doomed mate. But some were messages of a more dangerous nature and, if allowed to fall into the wrong hands, could ultimately threaten the safety or freedom of the sender. These messages the child had learned to commit to memory; leaning close to her recipient's ear, she would close her eyes and recall, without error, the message, how and from where she had received it. She had become so adept at memorizing and repeating them – able to repeat them verbatim – that with time she became for the internee their little spy from the outside world.

But today, she had to work harder to concentrate on her chores as the voice of that dark new arrival caught her attention. His tones were so strong that they caused a resonance inside her like when she was close to the big bells of Notre Dame. He was now in deep conversation with M. Verginaud and M. Valeze, whom she deduced he must know quite well from the warmth of their laughter, the freeness of their gestures and the fervor of their elaborations. She wanted to get closer. She noticed that the stranger's wall was lined with many more books than she'd seen among the others and that he had a good cache of writing paper stacked on his pallet.

"Where's mine?" barked the very gaunt man lying near her. His harsh summons alerted her back to her duties. M. Pierrot was one of the few here the child tried to avoid. No matter how meticulously she tried to satisfy his demands, he always found a way to be dissatisfied. Twice a week she brought him sweets, a gift from his equally disagreeable daughter. No matter what the weather, the child would be left to wait outside M. Pierrot's home while his daughter put together a puny package of sweets, which she thrust through the door, and then slammed it in the child's face.

"You've stolen some of my sweets! You little beast!" Pierrot shook the battered box at her. In fact, she had taken to stealing one or two of the caramels as commission, figuring that Monsieur would never notice his daughter sending so few anyway. But today the box had been badly crushed by the heavy volume of things she was delivering to M. Champeneux. "This is trouble." She was not pleased.

"Here, sir," she said sheepishly, but without apology, extending the box to Pierrot while keeping as much distance between them as she could.

"You filthy wretch, miserable daughter of a whore!" Pierrot screamed, leaping to his feet, his long taut frame rigid with rage. She tried to step away from him but he caught her by the wrist. "I'll teach you to steal from me!" he said shaking her and squeezing her hand so hard the box flew up then crashed to the floor sending all the caramels scattering. "You'll learn some respect, you whelp of a bitch!" His hand flew up and she covered her head with her free arm waiting for the blow to land.

"That will be quite enough, my friend."

The girl recognized the dark stranger's voice. She peered over her arm to confirm his presence and saw that he had caught M. Pierrot's forearm mid-swing, like a vice, in his large, powerful hand. Immediately she was released. The stranger spun M. Pierrot and, with a contemptible shove, forced him firmly back onto his pallet.

"I've saved you, friend, from a grievous error," the man said to Pierrot, flashing his dark, intense eyes at the child. She could have sworn she saw sparkles of light burst in them as he acknowledged her.

"You thought you were going to teach a lesson by brute force or injury to this little cur, this gross inferior to your magnificent self. But you Monsieur, are quite misguided. I can see that. First, because you find it necessary to threaten one whom anyone can see is not your physical equal. And secondly, because you are unaware apparently that this miniature redheaded moppet is our special lifeline to the outside world."

By now he had attracted most of the other prisoners who formed a ring around the scene.

"I'm distressed, sir, to see that it never crossed your mind that she might be made of far rarer and finer stuff than we. I am not wise enough to know whether she be an elf, sylph or leprechaun, but I clearly see she is a magical creature and, as any fool knows, to harm a representative of the fairy kingdom is to invite disaster upon one's head."

By the affirmation and solid chuckles of the others, the child began to feel quite the outstanding figure.

"Indeed, my friend, I have probably saved you and us all from a most horrible fate, which in your selfish, self-satisfying state you have completely disregarded. Look at her, this tiny button of a thing, dirty, disheveled, hungry, someone anyone would assume is an object to be pitied or scorned. But, friends..."

His voice had risen to a strong, melodious rhythm. The child craned to watch every facial gesture of her hero. He extended his arms, his white shirt sleeves billowing.

"Look about you at these thick, sweated stone walls, windowless but for the small air holes just wide enough to accommodate the rats. Who among us, the brave, the articulate, the strong, can pass in and out of these walls at will, as if they were mere spun sugar? Only she!"

He brought one long arm down in her direction and held his palm open to her.

"Yes, only this one, my friend!"

He turned to Pierrot, whose expression had gone from indignation to disbelief.

"Had you struck her, had you harmed her, only God knows the sort of revenge she and her legions would have chosen for you. Perhaps she would have made you a toad."

He crouched a bit closer to Pierrot's now blank face. Everyone laughed at the game.

"Or maybe she'd make you disappear, or worse yet." He bent close to the ear of Pierrot, his whisper far too loud to go unheard. "She might have you called to the guillotine with tomorrow's sun! I may have intervened just in the nick of time and Monsieur, perhaps if you were to proffer a heartfelt apology, rather quickly I suggest, since these ones are generally short on patience, I am sure in her graciousness she will accept and bear you no threat of malice."

"ABSURD!" Pierrot said. "I will never apologize to that trash. And who are you?" he demanded.

The child stopped marveling, the practical side of her locking in. Yes, she wanted to know this too.

"I am General Francisco de Miranda!" the man said. "And you my poor fellow are a disappointment. I thought you'd see it, but I now understand that you don't at all."

"See what?" Pierrot asked.

"You are stone blind to what stands before you? She is Pandora, child of Zeus and Minerva. She is the bringer of all things!" In a sudden flash of movement Miranda had taken Pierrot off his pallet and twisted one arm behind his back. He pushed it up against the shoulder blade and Pierrot winced.

"Miss Pandora," the general said, addressing the truly startled girl. "Will you accept a sincere apology from this wretched bully or no?"

She was paralyzed by all this attention—never had there been such a fuss over her. The general prodded her by nodding yes, behind the back of the grimacing Pierrot. The child followed his lead.

"We are in luck! It isn't too late!" Miranda said. "Now sir, repeat after me." He cinched up Pierrot's arm a notch.

"Mademoiselle Pandora," Pierrot repeated after Miranda, "please accept my apology."

Miranda exerted a little more pressure on the reluctant man's arm and his voice immediately hit that high, tight level which evoked laughter from the audience. "Please accept my apologies," he repeated again with just the right mix of sincerity to prompt the child's brusque "I accept."

"You are indeed a lucky fellow," Miranda said, giving the bruised malcontent a solid thump on the shoulder.

"As my friend is a bit shy and short-tongued," Miranda said, "I am sure he would want me to present you with these as an added gesture of his regret."

Miranda picked up some fallen caramels and presented them with a flourishing bow. "Mademoiselle Pandora, sweets for the sweet."

CHAPTER FIVE

The child had donned her new name as joyfully as a robin welcomes a new spring. Now, each day as she made her way to La Force, the yearning to hear it said by one and all propelled her through her errands and hastened her arrival, sometimes getting her to the gate before the evening guards had changed over their shift. This gave her the extra, "Good morning Mademoiselle Pandora," from both sets of guards. Haly and Mathilde had accepted it too, though somewhat begrudgingly. "Well at least we know who we are talking to," Mathilde snorted one day when Pandora had taken offense to the old appellation of, "Come here, girl."

"It's a grand name," she told Ravage, with serious formality. "If you should hear someone calling 'Pandora! Pandora!' as is apt to happen, you should know it is me who is being called. It is a very old name with a special meaning, the 'bringer of all things'," she explained to the black mongrel. "The general himself gave it to me!" Ravage had cocked his big bony head curiously accepting her earnest scratching behind his ears.

But the general had become the primary reason for her haste each day to La Force. Ever since his arrival, everything in her life had changed. With every visit she brought another tool by which the striking-looking soldier kept his mind keen and his spirit alive. Mostly they were books which he had instructed her to find in a small book shop, secreted away in an alley behind the markets of Les Halles. Writing notes on his fine watermark paper, Miranda would explain to her the exact volume and edition he desired. At first, in an attempt to impress him, she pretended to understand the script on the papers he handed her by nodding knowledgeably. The general, knowing full well that this was a ruse, joined in the game by reading aloud all required information. But he did it quickly and without pause as a private test of the child's prodigious memory. Thus the two played out their hands.

Those bound pages she brought soon assumed a monumental importance to her and General Miranda always rewarded her journeys with a generous gratuity earmarked for a specific purpose.

"Here, now," he'd say. "This is for a good bowl of stew." Or on another occasion, "Here, this is for some cutlets and cheese, and this for a hair comb." Pandora followed these instructions to the letter like all the others. But her biggest thrill was not the material reward she received from him. It was the readings. Every time, after her rounds of the room were done, Miranda would sit her down on his pallet and read to her.

The idea that the bewildering black marks that adorned these pages could be transformed, through his sonorous voice, into images such as red fruits, trees bent to the ground from a furious wind and rain, or a sailing ship becalmed on a vast green sea was to her no less than magic. In her mind's eye she could picture these places she had never been, nor even suspected existed.

As it became increasingly important for the child to gain entry, she was more and more obliging toward the turnkey and his wife. At painful cost, she would bring Mathilde fresh pastries filled with rich vanilla cream and sometimes covered with caramel sugar. Mathilde, having quite a taste for sweets, showered much kindness on her when she arrived with these treats. But Haly's demand was of a different sort, and Pandora nourished this well. She would pretend to carry from within the prison elaborate compliments and declarations of respect, which she claimed to have overheard while making her rounds. Haly would laugh greedily as she told him of the prisoners who spoke of how "powerful and respected" he was among them, and often he would punctuate these affidavits by puffing himself up and pointing a crooked finger at Mathilde, saying, "You see how they speak of me? You see the force within which I stand?" Then, because he was insatiable for this praise, he would send the child back into the inner prison, calling her "his little spy" and advising her to keep her eyes and ears sharp while moving about.

Today, with her little satchel heavy, she sailed along at a brisk pace, ignoring her shortening breath, which demanded she slow a bit. The treasured book she carried this morning was of her favorite sort and she'd lingered a bit longer than usual at the bookseller's narrow reading table, inspecting with care the drawings of strange and magnificent creatures within. So, despite her load, she pressed on energetically.

Of late, her trips to La Force had been as close to idyllic as she could know. There had been a respite from the calls to the guillotine, which lightened everyone's mood as well as hers. One of Pandora's most unpleasant and unprofitable errands was having to tell the families of those selected for execution about their fate. But the lull in morning selections had made her access easier and she came and went as she pleased. Often staying far into the evening, she would find a place a respectful distance away and with total concentration she would study and listen to General Miranda. He spoke of many important matters with the others, his strange accent filled her with secret imaginings about his homeland and his brave deeds. She studied his gestures, wide and strong. At times she even tried to extend her arms the way he did, as if embracing everything in sight. She watched as he paced with a military erectness. She marveled at his thick dark hair, and admired how he held his quill and tilted his papers when he wrote, the way he crossed his right leg over left when he sat reading to her. In short, she became so engrossed in his very being that she gave up her flower selling in order to spend every possible moment in the circle of her champion.

Even before she darted across the last bend of the boulevard a terrible darkness overtook her bright anticipation. She heard them, the shrill raucous cries of the women who went from prison to prison clogging the gates with their numbers, screaming for blood, for revolutionary justice, for heads. These overzealous hags always meant trouble of the worst kind—they were the harbingers of the blade. Pandora knew with seasoned clarity the brief holiday had ended and another torrent of blood was about to begin. A sudden knot of panic propelled her to the gate. She had to get inside. If the lists had been brought last night, her general's name might have been on it. No matter what, she had to get through that gate, immediately. She pushed into the crowd stomping on toes, jabbing with her elbows, pinching, even taking up the cry of the rabble. Hopefully she would win entrance because of her familiarity, but when she had finally managed, sweaty and disheveled, to reach the gate, they were bolted shut and the guards had stationed themselves in front with their backs to the street.

"Gendarmes!" she cried. "It's me, Mademoiselle Pandora, the messenger! Please, I must go inside, M. Haly needs my assistance! M. Gendarmes, please, it's me!"

It was to no avail; they didn't even turn to see who called to them. She tugged on the sleeve of a small, sinewy woman whose neck muscles and veins stuck out from the effort of her screams.

"Have they brought the carts?" she shouted. "Have any been taken in?"

"Blood! Death to the traitors!" the woman chanted, jumping up and down, knocking Pandora about. Suddenly, her books, her messages, her papers all seemed a ton of weight. She forced her way out of the frenzy and sat down across the street to wait and watch.

Surely there would be activity soon. Perhaps she'd be able to sneak in when the carts came to deliver new prisoners and, once inside, maybe she could skip her stop at the turnkey and go right to the big room.

As the hours passed and the sun moved to high noon, Pandora did not stir one iota. She kept all her focus on the prison gates. Suddenly, she heard the roll of wheels coming from the boulevard and soon she saw three carts with new prisoners heading towards her. Immediately the women turned their malice on the approaching caravan. Picking up stones and trash, they dashed from the gate crying, "Death to all aristocrats! Off with their heads!"

Pandora ran towards them. Phillipe was nervously leading the line. She pushed her way to his cart, grabbed onto the small ledge at its back and hoisted herself onto it, pulling her precious satchel after her, securing it between her curled legs. The frenzy of the women grew even greater—they hurled trash, which splashed on everyone, including Phillipe and the other drivers who reined their carts close together as they gained on the entrance, thus hiding Pandora well between the first and second cart. Then she heard

Ravage's growls. From her hiding place she saw him chained at Haly's side just inside the gate. They were backed up by more guards, their pikes at the ready. "Move ahead!" Haly ordered Phillipe. Pandora heard the gates open and the sound of the straining, slobbering dog held tight at the collar by his master. The guards charged the women, splitting open a path for the entering carts, which lurched awkwardly at the slow pace and their close proximity to one another. When Pandora heard the gates slam and the bolt slide and saw the guards retreat to their posts, she jumped from her hiding place and scooted quickly to Haly's office, arriving there just before him.

He was clearly not happy to see her when he came, snapping Ravage's chain harshly from the dog's massive neck, the saliva hanging in strings from its open and working jaw.

"You'll have plenty of work tonight," he said, turning his back on her. "Quite a load of evening mail there'll be."

Pandora sickened. They hadn't been called yet, the time was coming. She hurried to the chamber, barely acknowledging the youthful guard who greeted her warmly.

"There is going to be a call tonight," she whispered to Miranda. She hadn't stopped at all even to put her satchel down. She just stood there looking up at him, her face hot, her cheeks twitching involuntarily, a precursor to the tears she fought valiantly to hold back. The general was completely calm, and smiled down at her warmly.

"Did you bring the book?" he asked.

She hesitated, his demeanor throwing her off. "Yes."

"Very good."

Pandora reached in her satchel and handed Miranda the book.

"It will serve us very well this evening," he said, leaving her and going off to converse with some others she'd noticed gathering about his pallet.

A palled silence engulfed the room, save the covered mumbles from Miranda's alcove. Pandora completed her deliveries with dispatch, anxious to sit near the general and wait for the coming "calls." The women had finally gone from the gates so that now, inside and out, nothing but the shuffle of a guard pacing the halls or the steady sighing of a fearful prisoner or a distant clang of another chamber door resounding about this cavernous place could be heard. For Pandora this time of waiting made everything about the chamber different. The very same light was grayer, gloomier. The faces of all, so familiar to her, were like dead, expressionless strangers. She wanted to throw herself at Haly's feet and beg his mercy to remove the general's name from the list if it appeared there.

Miranda alone proceeded to his business as usual, making notes, conversing quietly with one or another comrade, or looking through the new book of Cooke's Travels which she had brought.

Then there was a loud clang of bolts moving, locks jamming back and footsteps coming down the nearest corridor. It was Haly. Pandora and the others heard the click of Ravage's paws keeping time with his master.

This was it. Everyone came alert. Eyes that had dulled became bright. Pandora's heart beat so hard her little frame began to tremble. She saw Haly's blurred eyes as the guard let him into the chamber. He wavered just a bit as his second put down the box on which he always stood to call out the names. Without ceremony, he began, "Marcel Pierrot, Hubert LaFosse, Robert Ledru!"

"This is it for this section," he said, hauling Ravage out by the collar as quickly as they came.

No sooner had the door slammed than Pierrot, her old adversary, ran to it.

"No! No!" he cried. "Not me. There must be some mistake, you didn't see it correctly. Come back! Come back!"

Pandora felt sorry, even though he'd been her tormentor, but her relief at Miranda's exclusion overwhelmed any sorrow she had for the others. Ledru, a heavy fellow, lay unmoved on his pallet. LaFosse began walking with ever increasing deliberateness in a small circle in front of his little section. Every now and then he ran his hand across the back of his neck.

Pandora stared at General Miranda who continued leafing through Cooke. For a time no one spoke. After a while Miranda rose, slowly, unfolding to his full height.

"Gentlemen, facing a known death is not easy. Nature in kindness shields us from knowing our time of departure, but man is far too cruel for this." As he was speaking he placed three chairs in the middle of the room.

"M. Pierrot," he called. "My friend, come and sit. M. Ledru, M. LaFosse, please come." He indicated the three chairs. Ledru and LaFosse, with obedient shuffle, took their places, but Pierrot had hidden himself in the darkest corner. He was leaning against the wall, one arm covering his eyes. Miranda walked over.

"Join us, M. Pierrot. It is a long time before dawn. There will be time enough for your thoughts."

His gentle manner soothed Pierrot.

"I am afraid and I am ashamed," he said, keeping his gaze on the floor.

"No one faces the blade without fear," Miranda said, guiding the submissive man to his chair. At this point everyone else, save de Chatelet, who could not walk, encircled the three doomed men and put their hands on their shoulders with a supportive cover.

"The three of you will leave tomorrow," Miranda began.

"And just as many have preceded you. So many more will follow—but let us not spend this night in fear and melancholia. Let us pass it instead with thoughts of glorious life, our lives, our adventurous lives, which, in their living, have stood for something and in their death will leave a consequence, a legacy full of wealth—not of the material kind, but wealth of the spiritual, full of purpose and manly courage, the sort that ennobles our species and remains for eternity. Most men do little with their short time on this earth, but that has not been true with those here in this room and we must not now let our barbarous tormentors rob us of all our rightful dignity when we walk to our end. We who have not yet been called, must help the others go from here with the honor and esteem their deeds have earned. After all, my friends, what is death but the beginning of another journey into an uncharted future."

Miranda picked up the new book.

"Our little friend has brought us *The Voyages and Adventures of Captain Cooke.*" Someone brought him a long candle.

"Let us steel ourselves through this difficult night with the legacy of another man's uncharted voyage. I believe it will give succor to you who stand at the edge of the abyss and help the rest of us who are right behind you.

"Sunday, October 8," he began, the candlelight shining bright on his face.

"Fine breezes and gentle weather, there is an opening on a beautiful bay."

All through the night Miranda read. Many candles were replaced, but no man slept nor wandered. The three doomed men remained firm in their chairs, straight-backed and stronger than when the general had begun.

At last came the sound from the long corridor of Ravage leading the rest. Pike carrying guards with dour faces marched into the chamber of silent listeners and flanked the three men, their expressions stern and efficient. At the door, Phillipe and Haly waited.

"Ledru, Pierrot, LaFosse, it is time," Phillipe said with emotionless authority. The three rose as strong and erect as they had sat all night. Miranda went first, embracing one, then the other, followed by everyone else in the room. It was a quiet and refined farewell, like guests at a dinner party each making sure to clink the final toast.

"Lead on, sir," Pierrot said, the first to the door. "We are ready."

Then he extended both arms around his two comrades and went out the door past Haly and Phillipe whose faces betrayed admiration and awe. The door slammed shut, the room fell dark save for one small wick, which burned obstinately on.

CHAPTER SIX

It was some time before the movement in the outside corridors abated and in the large room the men returned to the pallets. Although no one knew for sure when the doomed of La Force reached the guillotine, nor what roars of vengeance rose up when the blade had fallen on their final moments, each seemed to have a sense of it deep in his gut.

Pandora, who had born silent witness to the night's events, forgotten by the rest, walked slowly to the three empty chairs still placed shoulder to shoulder in the center of the room. She sat in each one and looked over at the table and the closed book from which General Miranda had read. She went over and methodically leafed through several pages of it and looked at the room from behind the table. Something was forming in her mind. She heard in her mind the general's voice even now in the dead silence. She took the book and sat cross-legged on a spot a small distance from his outstretched figure. She watched him with a penetrating gaze. She bore into him so deeply with her unblinking stare that it was not long before Miranda opened his eyes.

"You are indeed far more magical than I'd imagined," he said. "You seem to live without sleep."

Ignoring his whimsy she slid closer to him to speak unheard by the others. The general looked hard at her sitting in a little knot, her face strong and determined.

"Excuse me, sir, I didn't mean to disturb you, but I have something to ask you that's so important I wanted to put it to you as soon as you awoke."

"So you were going to sit there and watch me sleep?"

"Yes, General, sir, I don't mind at all."

Miranda sat up and lifted his eyebrows, a sparkle of delight softening his fatigued face.

"Then out with it, little one. Unburden yourself so we can both see to our rest. It has been a long night."

"Well you see, sir, it's like this. Even though I am very small, I really can do a lot of things. I am very good at messages, and if people speak clearly they need not write down a word. I can stick it in my brain and carry it to and fro without dropping a sound. I am also very good at getting in and out of places, and since people ignore me mostly, I can sit like a spider on the wall and take it all in."

She drew closer to him and whispered.

"I could be a very good spy." She looked at him anxiously awaiting a response.

"All you say is true, Pandora, but the point eludes me."

"You see, sir, I want to be yours. To work only for you. It wouldn't cost you very much. I could be like one of your soldiers, I wouldn't disappoint you. Believe me, I'd be worth my wage."

"This is indeed a serious proposal you've made, child, and if I were to agree there would be certain stringent conditions which would have to be met."

"Oh, anything you say, sir. I know there are lots of rules in the army."

Miranda smiled. "Well, first off, there's the matter of your quarters. Where do you live?"

"Under the Pont Neuf."

"Do you have family?"

"No, sir, none that I know of."

"Ah well, you see, there we have our first problem. A soldier can't live just anywhere. A soldier must have proper quarters. But if I were to accept you as part of my army, you could move into my home on Rue Menilmontant. There is a wonderful woman there named Francoise Pelicián, she is my housekeeper and she could see to your proper clothing and rations. A soldier must always be dry and well fed, you know. But, you are too attached to the open air life."

"Oh, no, sir!" she said. "Living in a house would be just fine for me."

"Then there is the very big problem of education. If you were to do any work in espionage, for which I agree you are well suited, there are languages which need to be learned. An ability to read and write. Mathematics, history. It's a great deal for someone as young as you."

"Oh, I can do it, sir. I may be small of limb, but if I may say so without seeming boastful, I have a very fast head."

"Indeed you do. Let me sleep on it, Pandora. Let us both sleep on it." He took his jacket from the straw and folded it like a pillow.

"Here, rest your head on this." Then he put his head down and closed his eyes.

"Oh, one more thing, General. I am not afraid to die."

CHAPTER SEVEN

As the summer sun began to set, Pandora crossed Paris from the prison to its outskirts. As she neared 17 Rue Menilmontant the light had almost disappeared. What little daylight remained bathed everything in that purple hue synonymous with dusk. The gray stones of the house reflected an iridescent rose-gold and as the child stood at the bottom of the steps, looking up at the triple-paneled oak doors, she surveyed her new home with exacting scrutiny. She noticed the roof of gray slate, each tile perfectly in place. Her keen eyes were drawn to the new mortar securing old stones and the brightness of fresh yellow paint adorning closed wooden shutters.

How could a man, she wondered, who had lost his freedom, keep (and keep so well) such a fine house? He must be very rich indeed. With a deep breath and determined stride, she marched up the steps, rose up on her toes to reach the lion's tongue of the black door knocker, and gaveit a sharp rap. No sooner had it struck its mark than the door sprang open and Pandora found herself looking up at a large woman whose bulk filled the entrance way. Her cheekbones were so high, such a remarkable feature, that one tended to gaze endlessly upon them and disregard the rest of her rough beauty. Her skin was drawn tight over her facial frame giving a most marvelous expression to every movement. The nose and lips were wide and full and her eyes seemed to shine with glistening clarity, the blue cores engendering the feeling of a wild bird. She looked down at the charge she'd been expecting and they both stood frozen. The imposing middle-aged woman in billowing skirt, her housekeeper's head tied in a scarf, the starched edges of which extended straight out to her broad shoulders, towered above the little ragamuffin. But in the next instant, Francoise Peliciàn broke into an enormous grin.

"You're not going to stand there and stare at me all night, are you?" she said. "Food for the belly, soap for the body, and a prayer for the soul—that'll fix you up right as rain." She swept Pandora inside and led the way to the kitchen. As they marched ahead, Pandora heard the rosary, which hung from her hip, marking time. In the cozy kitchen Francoise had set on a long, oiled-to-a shine, wooden table, a pitcher filled with milk, a plate of bread and cheese, and a bowl of raisins and hazel nuts. A high-backed chair stood in front of the repast waiting for its occupant.

"Sit," Francoise ordered. Pandora obeyed immediately, sitting on the edge of the chair, hands in lap, her eyes wide on the milk. Francoise poured a glass and stood on the child's right, crossing her fleshy arms over her large bosom. "Go on, child, go on. There's nothing I hate more than a reluctant eater." Pandora took up the cup with both hands and drained it in haste, swallowing hard and quick. Francoise smiled and poured her another cup.

"Good, you're catching on already. Action! Action is the key to life. You have many things to learn, and I am just the one to teach them to you." She continued pouring Pandora cupful after cupful as the child devoured each at a speedy pace.

"You seem to have quite a taste for milk, although I suspect it has been on rare occasions that you have had any."

Pandora was feeling more comfortable now, and the steady filling in her stomach with this fine drink helped her to speak.

"I only had it once before—a man in a bar bought my flowers with a pitcher of milk. He was drunk. He bought a lot of blooms, and I drank a lot of milk." Draining yet another cup, she announced, "I prefer it to wine."

Francoise exploded with a laugh that sounded like the trumpet call of a charge of hussars. Then she pushed the plate of food toward Pandora, coaxing her to move on to it.

While Pandora ate Francoise watched her closely, very much the way a mother does a baby as it learns for the first time to pull itself up on its feet, with a certain anticipation that the babe will fall and a strong regard for its tenacious efforts. When it became apparent that Pandora could not stuff herself with another morsel, Francoise drew her away from the table.

"Let me show you your room now. Then I shall bathe you."

As they went upstairs to the top floor, the child glimpsed a home of comfort. Each room was neat though simple and everywhere there were books. In fact, it was not unlike the bookseller's shop where each corner was arranged for the comfort of reading any of the volumes chosen. A twinge of excitement went through her as they ascended the narrowest of stairs and Francoise pushed in the door to Pandora's room. The first thing she saw was a small wooden bed with a light blue down cover over it. Francoise had lit the candle and the evening breeze, which blew in from the open dormer windows, caused the flames to dance merrily on the sloped ceiling. On the wall over the bed hung an old wooden crucifix.

"Mademoiselle Peliciàn," Pandora said. "It can invite much trouble to have the cross in one's home. I have seen many make the sign in secret so as to be safe."

Francoise looked at her squarely. "Now you listen to me, little girl, a choice between safety for the moment and eternal damnation is no choice at all. My mother died a good Catholic woman and so will I." Crossing herself with a bold and defiant gesture and bringing her face close to Pandora's, she pointed her finger as if the child were the object of her ire and said in deep tones, full of throat, "And may Robespierre burn in Hell!" Then she immediately set to work removing Pandora's old clothes.

Soon all of the little girl's filthy rags were piled in a heap on the floor, and Francoise wrapped her naked and dirty body in a soft robe. Pandora's senses were overwhelmed. The feel of clean cloth, the satisfaction of a full stomach and the comfort of a real bedroom were too much to absorb all at once. By the time she had been led back to the kitchen, where Francoise placed her in a wooden tub filled with hot water, those feelings were quite strong. They were beyond pleasant or unpleasant. They made her feel as if she were another creature in another world, one whom she did not yet know, but with whom she was acquainted. And indeed, as Francoise brushed and pulled the last tangle from her now shining red hair, Pandora looked like another child.

"Now it is time for a good rest," Francoise said, as she tied back her hair with a striped ribbon.

"Go and acquaint yourself with your bed while I burn your old things and clean the washtub."

As Pandora entered the room, the quiet struck her first. Never before had she slept in a place where the loudest noise was the muffled beating of the curtain weights against the window sill. She walked slowly around the room, touching the porcelain wash stand, the little upholstered chair and the night table. With each round she moved a little lighter and faster until she was skipping briskly from object to object; then she dove onto the down covered bed and watched the shadows on the ceiling until sleep overtook her. Francoise Peliciàn crept in past the child, blew out the candle and left Pandora wrapped in her blue cocoon.

The silent shift in the night wind fingered Pandora's bare shoulder as the somnolent child moved fitfully about, trying to place herself in a protected corner of the bed away from its chill. Pulling her arms in under her night clothes, she pressed them hard to her chest and drew her knees up, tugging the smock over her exposed feet.

But it was not the night chill which was disturbing her sleep; it was her persistent nocturnal terror pulling her from safety and comfort back to the Pont Neuf. The dream demons, obliterating the security of her room, reached with icy fingers into her maw, dragging her unwilling ghost right back to the quay and throwing her down onto the cold, hard stones. The benign sound of the weighted curtains tapping against the window frame played on the strings of the furies' harps, turning them into the banging of the box strapped to the back of the man most feared by the little orphans of Paris, "L'homme de la boite."

This serpent of the state roamed the streets with his dreaded box, its chain beating out his approach with rhythmic foreboding. When they heard it, the tiny voices of the children would cry out with warning, "L'homme de la boite, L'homme de la boite!" their echo ringing from street to street as they flew with fear in their eyes, tongues hanging out like dogs in search of a sanctuary—a sewer, cellar or empty crate—any place would do, and if none were near, they just ran with all the life that was in them.

The man with the box soon found he was no match for such

keen and wary youth, so he began to hunt at night, his banging chain the only foretelling of his presence. He would snatch them up swiftly in their sleep, depositing the unlucky ones inside the box. Then off he stalked in search of another, for the crate was capable of handling two—three if they were small. He carried them to the poorhouse where "L'homme de la boite" was paid by the head. If by chance one little one had not survived the journey, its corpse was dumped into the Seine, whereupon "the man" returned to the streets to earn his grimy bread.

Nothing held more terror for Pandora than "L'homme de la boite," even though she was past the age of his concern. The thump of the innocent drapes transformed by her dream caused her to cry out in a high pitched tone, "L'homme de la boite, L'homme de la boite!" Her feet began to run and her arms to flail about until her cries brought Mademoiselle Peliciàn rushing to her bedside.

Grabbing Pandora into her sturdy arms, Francoise Peliciàn drew the child close to her breast and wiped her brow, moist from her phantasmic flight.

"Sssh, poor baby," she said, rocking the whimpering girl. "It's all right, my child, you are here with me, in a clean and safe home, in a house which loves God and all that is decent. In His infinite mercy He has sent you to me and I will serve you as your mother would have wished."

Pandora clung tight to Mademoiselle's nightdress, her chimera remaining so fresh and lucid it was impossible for her to believe it had only been a dream. She looked around and sniffed the air for the scent of the river while her keen ear listened for the sounds of the street, until at last the continued prodding of Mademoiselle Peliciàn's gentle hand pushing her curls away from her face and the warm pressure of her lips pressing against her tightly closed eyelids summoned her away from her cold fright.

CHAPTER EIGHT

From her years under the bridge, Pandora was by necessity a fitful sleeper and never needed awakening. So as soon as Mademoiselle began to stir about in her bustle of predawn activity Pandora would be up and dressed. This unassuming event had quickly become a bone of contention between the iron-willed housekeeper and the free-spirited girl. Peliciàn had inflexible notions of the proper way to raise a child – she insisted that washing and a morning prayer be recited before anything else was tended to. So it was that Pandora was made to undress, wash, dress again and say prayers under the watchful eye of Mademoiselle before she was allowed to sit at the table for her bountiful breakfast of berries, bread, honey and milk, with a flavoring of coffee.

Her books were always stacked and ready for her departure to the prison of La Force where she had now become the mascot, the pet, the raison d'etre, the cause célêbre of all the inhabitants of the special room. Everything had been so meticulously tended to that Baron de Guiche, one of the newer prisoners, even dispatched his carriage and driver to pick the child up at seven a.m. sharp every day to bring her for her lessons.

General Miranda, having become the undisputed leader of this room, had used the education of the child as a way of giving life and purpose to all the prisoners, young or old, and all of them had risen to the challenge with unrestrained enthusiasm. The arguments and exchanges of ideas and pedagogical techniques which transpired between readings of the evening's "mail" and the next lessons were heated and fraught with debate, but their complete sense of purpose made this "faculty", in a university of one, a group unmatched. Miranda had carefully divided the curriculum, matching each man's expertise with an area of study. The walls became like great slate boards, filled with geometric diagrams, maps and paragraphs of writing in languages from Latin to English. Pandora's errands were curtailed and her driver kept a steady supply of candles and writing materials coming through. Haly and Mathilde, not being blind to the activities, were well bribed to secure Pandora's steady attendance for as many hours as required each day. As for Pandora, the excitement was intoxicating—from the warm milk and coffee in the morning to the last sentence etched on her slate at her little desk under the sloped roof at night.

She was numbed by the learning at the prison, and her insatiable craving served the others as completely as they did her. She knew well the function she played and understood she was giving these men as much as she received from them. She never wavered in her earnestness of practice nor her meticulousness of detail, and her progress delighted everyone to a state nearing ecstasy. Her youthful exuberance infected so, that if one was called away by the "mail", three more leapt up to take his place. The mutual devotion that flowed back and forth under the conduct of the general was close to miraculous. The only times when the tempo established by the general halted were at the "calls" from Haly and when Pandora returned home, exhausted but giddy, to Rue Menilmontant and Mademoiselle's waiting meals and discipline.

That night Pandora remained late, working with de Chatelet on her English. Miranda had made him chairman of the language department, and they had both decided the child should learn English and Latin. Despite the general's ministrations, the poison from de Chatelet's wound worsened his condition everyday, but his new responsibilities rallied his spirit and renewed his toughness.

"I go, you go, he goes, we go, you go, they go," she repeated, scratching the foreign words onto her slate. "Continue," de Chatelet said, resting somewhat shakily on his elbow, unable to sit straight.

The door opened and Haly, accompanied as always by Ravage, came in slamming the box onto the ground. Everything stopped as usual, but for some reason, as Haly stood up on the box and cleared his throat, de Chatelet whispered to Pandora, "Continue, child, let us not waste any time."

"Achille de Chatelet!" Haly read loud and clear, then in his regular hasty manner, slammed the door upon his exit. All eyes turned to de Chatelet and his pupil, Pandora's hand faltered on the slate.

"Continue," de Chatelet said.

"I am going, you are going, he is going," Pandora's voice echoed in the silence.

"Excellent," de Chatelet said, reaching over to her on the stool and squeezing her hand with his.

"We are finished for today, child. I have worked you hard and you have met the task. Perhaps when you speak this tongue in the future, you will occasionally remember me with fondness."

Pandora blinked very fast and smiled broadly at de Chatelet to mask her discomposure.

"M. Champaneux," de Chatelet said. "I am going to appoint you my successor. Come, we shall go over the future work together."

Champaneux came and sat with de Chatelet.

"General Miranda, sir," he called. "May I have a word with you when we are finished? I need to ask a favor."

Laced by tenderness and compassion, Champaneux formally discussed with de Chatelet Pandora's future in linguistic studies.

"The order of declensions must be in perfect sequence," de Chatelet said. "Watch her lip formations and listen carefully when she reviews her vowel group pronunciations in English. It is essential that the child be viewed as a person of elegance and background when she speaks."

"I will follow these rules as precisely and persistently as you have, sir," Champaneux said. "And we can count on the general to be a diligent overseer and make sure I do not slip from your standard of excellence."

Miranda and de Chatelet laughed at Champaneux's good natured jibe.

"Well now, General," de Chatelet said. Miranda pulled up his stool at the address. "M. Champaneux will be a fine substitute. The child is in excellent hands." De Chatelet pushed himself forward on his pallet, his festered leg horribly inflamed, causing excruciating pain with the least motion.

"May I help you sit," Miranda asked.

"No, sir, sitting is impossible. I am in need of a far greater assist right now, though I have the deepest regret that I must turn our conversation from the pleasurable importance of Mademoiselle Pandora's future to the irksomeness of my brief one. But there are two matters to which I must attend and I am embarrassingly incapable," he indicated his leg and near prone position, "of taking care of these myself. I regret imposing on our friendship in asking, but I must. M. Champaneux will you be my scribe and take down my last will and testament? And General, sir, will you be signatory as it is necessary for validation?"

"Certainly, we will," Miranda said.

"Very well, now, General, I have listened to you speak of your past and the hopes of the future. I will not be lucky enough to see yours nor that of my pupil, but at least I have a chance to choose my death. It is not that I fear the guillotine or the torturous pain which the movement of the journey to the Place de L'Execution will cause me. My fear is that the indignities of the jeering mob are beyond my strength of soul, and I am asking you to help me secure my final liberty by arranging a painless and clean death. I trust, given your wide experience, you are capable of providing such an end for me and that you will consent to do so." Miranda took de Chatelet's cold and bloodless hands in his and nodded assent.

"I will not balk, dear friend, at such a request. Many have chosen your course as a way to deny the savage hordes a final pleasure. I will prepare a 'medicine' for you immediately. We will fulfill your desire quickly, cleanly, and without pain, whenever you say the word."

"Thank you," de Chatelet said, beckoning both Champaneux and Miranda closer.

"Now," he said, a shade of relief in his tired eyes, "I think you gentlemen will both agree, it will be easier to achieve my first request before the second."

Miranda held a candle stump over the pages while Champaneux began to write the words dictated by the wounded soldier.

"In the event that my beloved wife Veronique should escape the terrible force of our present evil, I wish to leave her, with loving heart, the bulk of my estate. To M. Champaneux I leave all of my papers and any books he may find of a scholarly interest which will aid him in the writing of his History of the Republic. To General Francisco Miranda, I leave the following books, those authored by Benjamin Franklin, Bousset and Hobbes. Also my cottage and a parcel of land on the River Loire. Should mercy not reign on you, dear Veronique, I then bequeath all of my property to General Miranda, to be disbursed as he sees fit.

"Lastly, having not been blessed by the joy of children, I wish to remember one small one who, in the final days of my life allowed me the momentary bliss of knowing such a blessing. I give, in fond memory, a copy of Cooke's Voyages, Young's Travels and The Voyages of La Honton to our little redhead whom in this place we call Pandora."

***

De Chatelet raised his hand toward Miranda, signifying he was finished and would sign the document. With the general's help he weakly endorsed the page. Champaneux and Miranda followed, signing underneath. Then, with some candle wax, they pressed the seal from de Chatelet's signet ring onto the bottom.

Miranda went immediately back to his section and from the trunk under his jacket retrieved a bottle of fermented wine. He poured some onto the copper base of his candle stick, catching it underneath with a dish, then let it sit.

"What are you doing?" Pandora asked. She had been waiting on his pallet.

"I am preparing a 'medicine' for M. de Chatelet, which will spare him the indignity of tomorrow's journey. He has fought a hard struggle and now that he knows there will be no reprieve, he will not let the villains of tyranny be satisfied at the appearance of his weak condition and pain. When they come for him tomorrow morning his soul will be far away and out of reach of their blood stained hands. Through the interaction of these chemicals, this 'verdigris' will take him honorably to his rest."

CHAPTER NINE

"May I have some more bread?"

"Please!" Mademoiselle Peliciàn finished for Pandora, crossing herself quickly.

"If you'd be so kind to at least take a breath after grace, God would be able to hear your words unhampered by the sound of your chewing," she added, passing the rich dark bread she'd baked the night before.

"And stop swinging your legs so or you'll churn that milk to butter. You can sit still long enough to be grateful to our Lord for blessing us with a hearty breakfast and good health one more day."

"Yes, Mademoiselle," Pandora muttered, sullenly. She did not see the point in all this "praying before eating" manners to say nothing of the "curtsy and primp" business she was put through by her protectress. Surely, all this washing and fussing was a waste of valuable time.

"May I *please* have a bit more honey?" she said, leaning heavily on the "please" to emphasize her learned obligation.

"A drop of genuine sincerity is worth more than a pound of false form," Mademoiselle said, her admonition irritating the child even further, prompting her legs to start their circular swing anew.

"Pandora!" Mademoiselle snapped, but just as Pandora thought she was about to reap another unwanted parable, they heard an urgent pounding on the cellar door. Mademoiselle bolted from her seat, Pandora fast at her heels. Rarely did anyone come through the secret basement tunnel during the day.

"Who calls?" Mademoiselle whispered, leaning close to the

door.

"A son of Liberty," came the sharp response.

"Sired by whom?"

"Freedom and daring."

"Henri," Mademoiselle said, swinging up the crossbar of the wooden door for her brother, whose coachman's cottage, which faced the street a block away, was at the other end of the tunnel.

"I've news," Henri said, winded and powdered with dust. "It's a great day, sister, a great day. They've risen up and caught the dragon himself."

"What are you saying?" Francoise asked.

"Shot him. He lays now, as I relate this to you, wounded, a condemned man, soon to have his head part his body."

"Praise be to our merciful Lord Jesus!" Peliciàn said, clutching her bosom where underneath she wore her crucifix.

"Now that his head will fall, so will this terror end," Henri said.

Pandora's comprehension of this news was as complete and enthusiastic as Mademoiselle and her brother's, but her first thoughts raced to her general. Did he know yet? She wanted to be the one to bring him the complete report. Robespierre, the general's enemy and persecutor, was soon to vanish from their lives, paying with his blood for his sea of sins. She must be a witness to all, to be his eyes and record without embellishment the entire story. This was her duty as his spy and soldier. Nothing else would do but for her to speed now to the Convention. How proud the general will be of her initiative and quick action. She grabbed a last piece of bread from the table, ignoring her beloved books for now, and scooted like a squirrel to the door, slamming it just as she heard Mademoiselle call out her name. Racing to the corner past her waiting carriage, she darted from one street to the next, using every shortcut she knew, her mind imagining how merry her news would make all the prisoners, but mostly she imagined the prideful gleam in Miranda's eyes as he retold for the others the exclusive report she was going to bring him.

When she arrived at the Convention a crowd was already gathered just inside. She dropped to her knees and wheedled and wormed her way forward.

"Ouch! You're on my hand!" she said to a man who'd stood

firm, preventing her forward thrust.

"Oh, pardon," he said, parting his legs to let her through. At the front she stopped still and looked up to see, lying unceremoniously across a large oval table with a green cloth cover, Maximilien Robespierre. Blood ran heavily from a wound in his jaw, onto his chin and white collar and spread in small pools onto the boxes on which perched his head. There was a lot of outcry from the gathered mob, but none moved beyond the line at which they'd stopped. The large gold embossed wall clock, its cherub-fashioned hands pointing the hour, struck 7 a.m. and from a distance as far as the Place de la Revolution, Pandora and the others heard the first calls for blood.

Spurred on by the gathering fury outside, those inside began to heap their jeers and insults onto the sky-blue clad figure struggling to upright himself. Pandora remained still, watching and listening, trapping everything into her steel memory. But her busy recording did not obfuscate deeper observation; she noted the irony of the situation as she looked about at the fierce faces spewing their vile cries of condemnation. Here were those same fools who'd so short a time ago sung the praises of the great Robespierre, now flaying him with their words.

Robespierre fussed and twitched about with his slim fingers, dabbing at the bleeding wound, then wiping at his jacket vainly, to remove the steady stain of blood. A nearly bald gaunt man with a sharp protruding chin came to him and began stuffing small pieces of paper into the gaping wound.

Two hours passed in a state of hold, then a commotion started on the other side of the room, a pair of doors flung open and two more men were brought.

"Saint-Just."

The crowd squealed, Pandora moved left to the wall and balanced herself on one foot at the top of a column pedestal for a better view. The second man was carried in on a stretcher, his body was twisted and crippled and on his head was a large hideously pitted and dried wound.

"Who is that, citoyen?" Pandora asked a man leaning on the wall next to her.

"Couthon," he replied, moving to the front of the line and picking up the catcalls. A surgeon followed the guards carrying the stretcher. Pandora saw one of the guards standing by Robespierre give a knowing nod to the doctor who immediately went to work preparing him for execution. Promptly he withdrew three loose teeth and with each extraction the rowdy crowd waved and roared. Then he took some linen and wound it securely around Robespierre's head and jaw, staying the blood from soiling his clothing further, but it quickly drew a circle of deep red around his jawbone. Robespierre remained calm during all the proceedings and, when the doctor had departed, he fastidiously attended his person, drawing his stockings up methodically, tucking them under his twill britches. Then he ran his hand up and down, making sure nary a wrinkle showed. Four gendarmes closed in and hoisted him aloft in an arm chair and brought him into the tumult of the Convention's revolutionary tribunal for a "trial".

Pandora ran, weaving her way into the hall close to the ground underneath the raised arms of the shouting, frothy crowd. The room was packed. Every conceivable space from floor to ceiling was occupied by an agitated citoyen. Pandora scanned the entire assembly. People leaned forward, shrieking unintelligible words, shaking with fury their hats, their neck scarves, even their small bewildered children, at the sight of the blue frocked man. "Justice" spoke rapidly. Pandora left at once from the same entrance she'd come and raced along the route from the Place de la Justice to the Place de la Revolution. Citizens already lining the route were held back by burly gendarmes and guards. When she reached the Place de la Revolution, it was already overflowing. People crammed window ledges, occupied the rooftops and sat on the ridge tiles, their feet dangling dangerously over the edge. Pandora searched for a spot in full view of the giant guillotine, its monumental silence now tantalizing the omnivorous crowd.

"Here ya go, wee one." One of the women hoisted the child up. There was a group of six—like matrons perched on makeshift bleachers. Each had her own umbrella to keep out either harsh sun or rain. From the sight of well worn pillows, a small stand with pitcher and chipped cups, along with a couple of coverlets, it was evident these women had secured this place long ago and kept it like an added room in their homes. Toothless and haggard from their harsh lives, they sat, gossiping in the afternoon sun, darning their socks, crocheting their doilies, sipping soup from the chipped cups, waiting, today as every other since the reign, for heads to fall.

"Sit here, girl," one said to Pandora, patting her lap. "It won't be long. Now, we'll have some fun."

The others cackled as Pandora went obligingly to the woman and sat firmly on her over-cushioned thighs.

Soon the wild roaring wave of the crowd caught up to them and everyone stood and craned down to see the coming tumbrel carts approach. The guards pushed and strained, threatening the more earnest spectators with the sharp tips of their pikes, to keep a path open for the procession. As it neared Pandora and the hags, a young, rather lithe woman sprang out of the throng and jumped over the cart carrying Robespierre. She clutched his forearm in her claw like fingers and reached up and over him with her other arm as if she were casting a spell upon him.

"Go down to Hell with the curses of all wives and all mothers!"

"To Hell, to death!" cheered the women surrounding Pandora. Then she heard them making a strange rhythmic hissing and clicking sound through their toothless mouths as the frustrated guards pried the little woman from Robespierre and flung her back to the howling mob.

As the tumbrel stopped at the foot of the guillotine, its long shadow fell sharply over the death carts. Pandora's heart pounded in her chest and ears. She felt inside her bones that indeed the death of Robespierre meant a great wind of change was coming. She stepped to the edge of her perch.

The guards lay Robespierre on the ground purposely in full view of the blade. He would be the last and would remain there to watch the others go before. First came Couthon the cripple, who cried out with impassioned pleas, to the joy of the crowd whose temper had reached that of a large, raucous circus audience, appreciative of its high spirited entertainment. The frustration the executioner had untangling the writhing figure and securing him to the plank serving as his final bed only sent those viewing into greater frenzies of laughter and huzzahs. Saint-Just, who followed, met only mild cheers. They seemed to be putting their energy in reserve for the last and choice event.

Finally, a full half hour after the others were dissevered and tossed onto the death cart and the sun shifted the shadow away from his prone figure, bathing him now in hot light, was Robespierre raised to his feet and brought to the bottom of the steps. The drums rolled as he ascended along with the great Cyclopean blade taking its position. At the top the executioner removed the sky-blue jacket and secured him to the plank. A silence of anticipation, one enormously held breath overtook the massive audience of Paris. Robespierre's head was placed in the blood drenched window under the poised edge of the blade. The executioner ripped the linen bandage from his face, and a cry, "Donnez moi la mort! Donnez moi la mort!" rose from the figure above and out over the silenced mass. The blade fell, the roar came with the power of thunder in a mountain storm. Pandora realized this villain, this bleeder of France, this dragon, was only a man and she jumped to the street and set her sights to the prison.

CHAPTER TEN

The following months taught Pandora a new kind of lesson. Right after Robespierre's death, she had thought it would only be another week or two before the gates of La Force would open for good, and all of her teachers would be freed and that General Miranda would climb with her one glorious evening into their carriage and return to Rue Menilmontant. But the machinery of justice moved at a much slower and more independent pace, affecting everyone in unpredictable ways.

Although the ranks of her professors began to thin as each secured his release, Pandora continued to come to the prison as before, books under her arm, her mind primed and eager for the barrage of facts, figures and ideas which were filling it. But the anticipation of freedom rather than the dark shadow of the guillotine had changed the mood in the big room and in her general. His energy was turned in a different direction. While it seemed his life force was still infused with the double-lightening that had previously been apparent, his prior occupation with philosophical ideas now turned to more earthly matters. Almost every evening now when she finished her lessons, she would sit and listen as he discussed with the others his "mission," which was the liberation of his native Venezuela from the Spanish Crown. He would spread maps out on his pallet and would engage any of the willing in debate on the various strategies he'd been charting. He would theorize on potential directions and comment on the great global changes he saw emerging, dwelling deeply on both the American and French Revolutions.

This "mission," of which Pandora now heard a good deal, had changed her position with the general. Although he did not ignore her per se, she became aware of a kind of matter-of-fact way in which he dealt with her. This gnawed at her and made her think that now that freedom was close at hand her importance was no longer as pertinent as his "mission." In reaction, she plunged with even more Promethean effort than before into her studies and eagerly brought the results of the labor to him and anxiously awaited the praise and approval he'd always given and to which she'd grown accustomed. But instead she was met with what she felt were cursory pats and praise.

He was preoccupied with other matters and she bottled her disappointment and hurried home to drive herself even harder on the next day's lessons. Finally, when Haly came and announced that General Miranda was to be freed and she walked with him into the bright fall sunlight, she was surprised that the long dreamt of sense of elation she thought she'd have was in fact a feeling of sadness and loss of the old times and their constant threat of disaster. She took General Miranda's hand as they crossed the road and climbed into the carriage and as they both watched the prison disappear from view, she was ashamed of her private feelings.

Mademoiselle Peliciàn was in a complete whirlwind with the general back in the house. In the first few days of his return, all her energies were spent on the maintenance of the home and Pandora became her assistant housekeeper.

"The house needs a scrub from top to bottom and you may as well learn what it's all about, so you'll know what for, when you have your own," she told her.

Reluctantly, Pandora obliged and ran from the market to the launderers, to the butcher, to the baker, never once being asked to stop at the old bookseller's and bring back a prize leaf. Her days were full of scrubbing windows, beating rugs, rolling dough for bread and aiding Mademoiselle in serving meals. She hated this change in status and, as the days passed to weeks, she became quieter and began to see herself outside the circle in which she'd been the center.

The house was full of visitors who came in a never ending stream through the secret tunnel. On any given night there could be anywhere from four to ten people sitting at the dining table. They spoke English mostly and all had a refined manner, but they were aware of Pandora's presence only as Mademoiselle's second and in this manner she was excluded from the conversations, which often went way into the night and which, just as in the prison, concentrated on the general's "mission." So after all the kitchen work was done, Pandora, whose English had become almost a second tongue, would sit at the top of the stairs and eavesdrop wondering why she was being excluded. After all, wasn't she still his soldier, a part of his army?

***

There was still suspicion surrounding the general and because of this, the house was under the constant surveillance of two gendarmes who remained conspicuously posted on the front steps, day and night. Mademoiselle's sense of Christian charity and astute nature had prompted her to ply these two watchdogs with plentiful food and drink, which Pandora was designated to deliver. She in her own way found that her quick wit and small stature charmed them as much as Mademoiselle's food, so between the two they'd kept the guards' attention diverted from any activity going on inside the house.

One night when there were no "guests," they finished their sweet and Miranda pushed back his chair to stretch out his legs and relax, Pandora seized the moment to gain his attention.

"Let's play the mystery game," she said.

In the prison they had often played this game as a device for her to use her exploding knowledge with imagination and today she had worked long and hard to find a mystery person whom she was sure would stump and impress the general.

"I am thinking of someone you'll never guess," she said, her desperation to hold his attention drawing her closer to him, waiting for him to take her on his lap as he sometimes did.

"I am sorry, little one," the general said, "but tonight I have important letters to write and then Madame de Stal is having a gathering which I must attend."

"But you promised we'd play soon, and it's already been a long time. It won't take very long, and I already have a stumper."

"The general said he couldn't play, Pandora," Peliciàn said. "Now run along and lay out his dark jacket and white shirt ruff, and when you're done with that you might show some attention to your own room. Last I saw, it looked like a windstorm had passed through."

The general winked and motioned with his head that Pandora should obey, but his easy manner was not matched by hers. Her face felt hot with hurt and anger and she turned brusquely toward the general's room.

"I'll read you a nice Bible story when you're all ready for bed," Mademoiselle called after her.

With mechanical diligence Pandora laid out the general's clothing then went to her room and put away her books, papers and quills and lay down on her bed. She had this terrible feeling of emptiness. Suddenly this wonderful room, full of all her treasured books, the implements of her future, seemed remote and inhospitable. Sadness and loneliness began to engulf her and, as she looked at the ceiling above her, she began to feel confined, trapped like the men in the prison. Everything around her felt too close, too tight. She shut her eyes and in the black void she grabbed snatches of a woman passing quickly into her view. It never froze, but Pandora knew it was her mother. She turned onto her side and tried to put the figure together, to see her hands, her eyes, her hair which surely was red like her own. But nothing took form except a thought, disturbing and powerful—she no longer belonged here. Whatever purpose she'd served the general before, she feared he did not need her as his soldier any longer and she was not going to be anybody's maid!

She heard Mademoiselle's voice bidding good night to the general and knew she'd soon be up. Quickly she climbed into her nightdress and got into bed.

"Are you asleep?" Mademoiselle asked, pushing the door gently.

"No, Mademoiselle."

"Are you feeling all right?"

"Yes, Mademoiselle."

"Are you quite certain?" Mademoiselle came in and pressed her cheek to Pandora's forehead, checking her for a fever. "I've never seen you away from your books this early. Is your stomach upset?"

"No, Mademoiselle, I feel fine. I'm just a bit sleepy, that's all."

"Well, this is a first—a night where you're not scolded to bed and the books wrenched from your hands!" Mademoiselle chided. "How about a nice bedtime read from the Bible?"

"No, thank you, Mademoiselle."

"Child, what is it? It's not like you at all to refuse a story. What is troubling you?"

"I'm sorry, Mademoiselle I just don't feel like hearing a story; my mind is too unsettled to concentrate."

"Indeed. But what could be so powerful to cause such an indisposition in one as hearty as you?"

Pandora suddenly felt weepy. She didn't want to answer because she feared she'd just start sobbing and blurt everything out.

"Tell me what it is, Pandora," Mademoiselle said, and Pandora hearing the gentle coaxing in her voice, attempted to answer.

"Oh, I was just thinking..." She swallowed a clot of sobs, trying to force their way up. "I was thinking how things have changed since the general has returned from prison. I am not saying in any way that I am not happy he's home and safe, but everything has changed so."

Mademoiselle began to stroke Pandora's head. Pandora knew there was no sense hiding from Mademoiselle because she always knew when there was an upset.

"It is true that there have been many changes since General Miranda returned and I can safely say there are soon to be many more."

Pandora pricked up her ears, startled at these implications.

"You see, a man like him cannot stay long in one place. Life for his type is a series of adventures with little rests in between. Why, in the years I have kept house for him, he has come and gone so often and unexpectedly, I usually have a place set for him at the table, just in case. It used to be unsettling for me, as it is for you now, but after I learned his ways and grew to admire and respect his purpose, well, then it became easier to adjust to the sudden changes and serve him as best I could."

"I must go wherever he goes and be of valiant service to him."

"You have been, child," Mademoiselle cut in. "He's told me often what a great aide you were to him while in prison and here your assistance to me and mere presence to him have been of unquestionable importance and pleasure. In fact, he was remarking to me of the way you've become a fine lady in these two years and, as a matter of fact, just this evening before he went out, we discussed at some length the future course of your education after the general departs."

The force of the last word shot Pandora upright, startling Mademoiselle.

"Pandora!" she said. "What is it?"

"You said the general is departing?"

"Why, yes, of course, just like he always does." Her voice was very calm and natural. "He has been planning to return to England and to his family there, to continue his plans. And that is why we were discussing your future."

Pandora did not know what to say first. What family was Mademoiselle speaking of and what future?

"Future!" fell involuntarily from her lips.

"Yes, darling. You have achieved so much, but there is more to learn before you become a proper young woman."

"But I do learn. I do study to the best of my ability, so I will serve the general as a good soldier, and spy, and be useful to him with his mission." Her sense of shock and fury began to rattle her composure, and she threw herself back on her pillows.

"Dear, girl!" Mademoiselle said. "Your head is so full of foolish notions. You are not a soldier, or a spy, but a fine young girl who has been rescued from a rough and unfortunate start."

"But I am meant to be with the general!"

Mademoiselle laughed kindly, but Pandora only heard it as painful ridicule.

"Child, right now you are meant to finish your education, and then we'll see to the general. There is a lovely convent school, The Sisters of the Sacred Heart, in the south, where I grew up. This is the place that will train you in fine fashion, smoothing all your rough edges and teaching you all you need to learn so that some day you will find a proper husband and raise a beautiful family."

She felt like Mademoiselle was sending her to the guillotine. How could this be? General Miranda had taken her as his own personal aide and now they were going to send her away and he was leaving as well, returning to his family! What was she? Certainly not family, not his soldier! All her observations had been correct. She was nothing here and now she had the proof.

"Pandora?"

"Yes, Mademoiselle."

"What do you say, doesn't it all sound lovely?"

"Yes, Mademoiselle." Pandora turned onto her side. "Lovely." Her heart turned cold as ice, and all the muscles in her little body clenched tight and hard.

"Well, we will talk about it some more tomorrow. Sleep peacefully, precious one."

"Good-bye Mademoiselle. I mean good night."

"You are dizzy tonight." She heard Mademoiselle chuckle as she closed the door.

Pandora shot out of bed and went straight to her writing desk. The moon had come round full and shone silver bright on the neat stack of papers and notes. She sat down, rod-straight, dipped her quill and began to write.

Dear General Miranda
and Mademoiselle Peliciàn,

From the very bottom of my heart, I thank you both for the kindness you have shown me and the things you have taught me. But it seems now that whatever usefulness I may have served in the past has expired and that I will become more and more of a nuisance or, even worse, a burden to you as time goes by.

With this in mind, I think it best I should be on my way and relieve us all of these worries. I hope you will not think that I am in the least bit ungrateful, for that is far from true and perhaps someday I will prove that to you with grand deeds.

Always your obedient servant,
Pandora

She folded the letter and placed it atop her books, weighting it with a glass paperweight. She began to dress, her face wet with hot tears.

CHAPTER ELEVEN

Back on the street again, Pandora was stimulated by the old familiar smells, rhythms and sounds. Fueled by her burning desire to show Mademoiselle Peliciàn and the general that she needed no one, her imagination flew to fancies of returning to them a grand success. She headed along the quay planning her strategy for employment and laughed at the image of herself submitting to the demands of some curtsy-conscious convent school. A job was the first order of business in establishing a foothold from which she could climb. Now that she was older and wiser, she certainly would find the right situation with dispatch and would not have to resort to her old ways and haunts.

She passed up the most likely places of employment—bakers, laundries and millinery shops, reasoning that a restaurant with a foreign clientele would be the ideal match for her skills and an employer's needs. So, with some well placed inquiries her trail finally led to a cozy restaurant, just off the main boulevard, which was frequented by an international set. This had to be ideal, she thought.

"Good morning!" she announced herself cheerfully, as she boldly strode inside. A man sat at a table with slips of papers strewn before him. His few remaining hairs were slicked back tight to his skull with some shiny oil, which reflected the tarnished light that illuminated his corner. There was a bar behind him with a carved mirror behind it. Several booths lined one wall, with maroon curtains separating one from the other, and opposite them were ten or so tables, their chairs at present set atop them.

"And the same to you," the man said, a preoccupation clouding his response.

"I can read and write fluently in English," Pandora said, "and my mathematics are flawless."

"To say nothing of your modesty," the man replied, smoothing his pate with a delicate hand. "If you're looking for work, I've none," he said rising, an invoice in hand, and going to a stack of boxes containing newly arrived produce. Pandora noticed several waiters now clearing the tables of their chairs and dropping piles of utensils and folded cloths onto them in noisy preparation for the days meals. She was unruffled by the proprietor's rejection and rather than heading for the door she brazenly walked to the table where his paperwork was laid out and scanned the bills. She was in luck, there was her meal ticket staring her right in the face.

"You know, of course, your butcher's bill is wrong and if you pay the requested amount, you'll have been cheated 10 sous."

"What!" the restaurateur exclaimed, leaving his produce to check on the horrid possibility. "I'll be damned if you're not right. How did I miss that?"

"Overwork," Pandora said.

"My name is Shapiro, what's yours?"

"Pandora."

"Pandora what,"

"Just Pandora."

"Well, 'just Pandora', I see you do have quite a head for figures and if your English is half as good as you say, perhaps I was a bit too hasty. Let me see what my wife has to say." The man grinned broadly, exposing teeth much too big for his circular plump face.

"Ethel!" he called toward the bar. A very petite, delicate, auburn haired woman came out from a mirrored door adjacent to the bar.

"What is it, Hermann?" she said, wiping her hands on her apron and pushing back a piece of her luxuriously thick mane, twisting it back into the bun and sticking it with one long thin hairpin.

"Come here. Come meet someone."

Pandora was delighted to see that the man's excitement was unmasked and if she could win the wife over she had herself a job. She focused on Madame Shapiro's sweet smile.

"Who is this?" Madame Shapiro said, looking down at Pandora with a special maternal warmth illuminating her face.

Pandora deduced she must have quite a brood of children. This will be an easy victory, she thought. If her deductions were accurate no real mother could resist her charm nor fail to empathize with her plight. Everything in this woman's expression told her that children were Madame Shapiro's soft spot.

"Twenty-seven times four?" Shapiro drilled Pandora, stifling a giggle like he was hiding a great surprise.

"One hundred and eight!" Pandora responded winking at him.

"Times that by 13?" he said.

"Fourteen hundred and four!" Pandora said, after a very brief pause to calculate.

"Why, this is incredible!" Ethel said, beaming with pride at her husband's great discovery.

"I'm thinking of taking her on. What do you say?"

"Well, there is no question, Hermann, this young lady will serve us very well." Madame Shapiro reached out her hand to Pandora. "Do you need lodging?" she asked, her kind nature flooding into Pandora's bones.

"Yes Madame if you don't mind."

Within the hour, Pandora had been given one of the small rooms in the back of the Lighthouse Restaurant, a modest wage, a black skirt, black leggings, white top and white apron complete with frill. She had begun her new job as a bar girl and assistant bookkeeper for this well-frequented establishment.

Pandora enjoyed her work enormously. She loved listening to all the different languages spoken and when she heard English, she was tickled ever so much at being able to respond in kind to the speaker. All of the patrons took to her from the very beginning and were especially impressed with how quickly she remembered their individual tastes. The Shapiros were equally pleased as ever and had no shame in displaying their pleasure toward her at any opportunity. Pandora had been right about them having many children, but none of them had survived infancy. Finally, they had found a child to put all their pent-up love into and how fortuitous that she be one as capable and special as Pandora.

One night Pandora noticed two men sitting in the darkest booth, their heads very close together, deeply embroiled in a conversation. They sat much longer than most customers and what attracted her attention further was that one of them, a fair, rather languorous fellow, seemed familiar to her. When she finally approached with their coffee and got a better look, she realized he was one of the Englishmen who'd come to Rue Menilmontant, through the tunnel. She stood a bit longer, studying him, waiting also to see if he recognized her, but he did not. His companion had jet black hair, very thick, wavy, well pomaded, and a tannish complexion. He was quite short, his belly bulged pushing the buttons of his vest to nearly popping. As Pandora turned away from the table she was sure she heard the dark man say, "Miranda." Furthermore his inflection was unmistakably Spanish, just like the general's—so she busied herself clearing the adjacent booth in order to hear more.

"Well," the Englishman replied.

"If you're going to get him you'd better move fast. I know he's planning departure for England very soon."

"Don't worry, friend," the dark one said, his gravely voice close to a sneer.

"Tomorrow morning I'm seeing a friend in a high position of the French government. The general's arrest for espionage is a surety. International intrigue is a deadly game."

Quickly Pandora took her dirty glasses to the kitchen, her heart beating hard, her breath short.

"Madame!" She tugged on Ethel's arm, which was immersed in flour. "I must speak with you."

"Of course. What is wrong? You're as pale as a sheet, child."

"Madame, you have been most kind to me and I will never forget you for it, but I have just overheard some distressing news, which will put someone very dear to me in grave danger. I did not want to run out of here without telling you, because it is not my intention that you should think ill of me. But if you will understand my urgency, I will return as soon as possible."

Without waiting to hear Madame Shapiro's reply, Pandora untied her apron and placed it in Ethel's flour-dusted hands. Then she ran out the door into the street, clutching her gratuities in her fist and jumped into the first cabriolet she saw.

"Seventeen, Rue Menilmontant!" she ordered, letting the driver see the color of her money. He struck the horse hard and headed in the right direction.

CHAPTER TWELVE

The driver of the cabriolet barely had the reins taut in his hands when Pandora demanded he stop a block from Rue Menilmontant. She jammed the coins into his waiting palm and jumped to the street. Under the ample shadows of the big trees which lined the side of the road, she snuck unseen to Henri's cottage. Putting her finger through the knothole of the loosened board she let herself into the basement and through the secret tunnel to the cellar of number 17. When she reached the kitchen door she stopped to listen. She heard Mademoiselle's footfall moving from table to basin. Undoubtedly, she was scrubbing the pots from supper or preparing the table for the morning as she always did the night before. She rapped the first bar of the signal and waited for Mademoiselle to approach.

"Who calls?" Peliciàn whispered sharply.

"A son of Liberty," Pandora responded, but before the next sequence of passwords could be exchanged, Pandora found herself held fast to the bosom of Mademoiselle. After a few moments enmeshed this way, she felt the force reverse and she was thrust back with the enormous strength of the woman's hands.

"I am not running a hotel, young lady. If you plan to use it as such, by coming and going of a free will, then you can stay away for good. I will not tolerate that kind of behavior."

"Don't put up such a thin facade, Mademoiselle." Miranda said from the doorway of the hall, then turned to look at Pandora. "The woman has been worried sick about you and has, I suspect, combed every street in Paris when I was not at home to prevent it."

"What I do, and where I go on my own time, is not subject for discussion and begs the point," Peliciàn said. "I will not cater to an ingrate." She turned full toward Miranda, giving Pandora her broad back.

"The child is a wild creature and I have failed to tame that streak. She quite plainly wants nothing of manners and Godliness, but only of the ruffian life. Look how she's already dressed in some low-class way, like a barmaid or what have you. Why, if she wants to submit to sin out there, that's not my affair." Despite this impressive bravura, Pandora could see that Mademoiselle had been truly distraught by her leaving. It surprised her.

After all, Mademoiselle was a strong taskmaster, what with her rules and manners and religion. Pandora had never let her resistance to them be hidden. That was why the two had so often reached a hard wall of stubborn resolve. She thought for sure her leaving would have brought the older woman relief. It was painful to see how deeply it had wounded her. However, enough of this thinking, the crisis at hand pressed.

"General Miranda, sir," she said, passing by Peliciàn, whose fuming and ruminations continued. "I've come back only to bring some news of great importance and distress." Behind her she heard Mademoiselle's lament cease as she settled onto her usual chair.

"What is it?"

As Pandora began to tell him of the blond Englishman and dark stranger she'd overheard, Miranda listened with acute concentration, his Spanish face set and stern. Meticulously she described the two men to him, recalling every conceivable detail. As she drew the faces with her words, she saw, in the general's expression, that she had again risen high in his esteem. She knew she had returned to her special position of regard.

"I know exactly of whom you speak," Miranda said, after she'd finished. "And he will be arriving here tonight."

"Tonight!" Pandora and Mademoiselle exclaimed simultaneously.

"Yes, we are making some final plans before my departure to England and, naturally, this spy in our midst would not be absent for the conclusion. But I have some conclusions of my own," Miranda said. "Pandora, once again I find myself deeply in your debt."

"You owe me no debt, sir. It is I who will never be able to repay you, I wish you God's speed and I hope this information has been useful." She turned to go.

"Pandora, please don't leave," Miranda said. "Given this sudden turn of events, if you are willing, I have one more mission, which I must ask you to perform."

Pandora turned. "If you ask, sir, I am always willing."

Miranda went and pulled a loose brick from the wall behind Mademoiselle's bread oven and counted out a quantity of paper money, which was hidden there.

"You remember the old bookseller behind Les Halles? Take this money and go to him now."

Pandora extended her hand and accepted the money.

"When you reach the back of the shop, knock on the door two times, count to three, knock four times, count two, then knock once more. When he asks who's there, you say, 'Diogenes in search of a lantern.' You will be admitted. Give him the money and tell him I need the papers for England tonight. He'll understand. Then return to me without hesitation."

Pandora absorbed all her instructions and pocketed the money. Again she turned to leave without acknowledgment or salutation.

"One more thing, Pandora," Miranda said, a warmer tone washing down that of his instructions. "I know that you are your own agent, so to speak, and while I disagree with your leaving, I do respect your desire for liberty. But I do think it advisable that you return to Mademoiselle and take the place we have secured for you in the convent school. I have left provision for you and, knowing more about the world than you do, I think it is a far more propitious course for you than the one you seem to have chosen."

Pandora had hoped, even assumed, he was going to ask her to join him. When he did not, she put her mind away from there and onto her task.

"I will consider it," she said. "I will return as quickly as possible and rest assured I will not fail you, sir." She ran down the cellar stairs.

By the time she reached Les Halles and hurried round to the bookseller's, all the streets were dark and deserted and her sweat chilled her body. She took a moment to review the code then proceeded directly to the first knock. After the proscribed series of raps, a candle flickered in a window above her. She watched it move from the room to the stairwell and approach the cracked front door.

"Who's there?" an anxious and tired voice called softly.

"Diogenes in search of a lantern." The door opened quickly and the old bookseller pulled her inside.

"Who sent you and what do you want?" he said checking the alley before shutting and bolting the flimsy door.

"Do you remember me, sir? It's Pandora."

The old man squinted and put his lantern close to her face.

"Ah, the runner for General Miranda. Indeed, yes. Well, I'd wondered where you'd been of late. Now what is it that brings you at this hour—must be of urgency to put you out at such a time."

"Yes it is," Pandora said, following the bookseller's scuffling steps down the slender hall to his shop. "The general has been betrayed and needs travel papers for England immediately." She was already taking out the money when they reached the shop and the seller lit his work lantern, checking the black shade over the front window first.

"Well, immediately, this is always the case isn't it? Caesar and Brutus, always the case." He blew the larger lantern out and picked up the smaller, then slowly headed toward the back room with Pandora in tow. Her agitation grew with each annoying delay. When they reached the back room, overstuffed with stacks and stacks of books, making precarious pathways all through it, Pandora felt the presence of someone else. She squinted about the smoky dimness and in a near corner she saw a man in priest's garb trying to conceal himself from her.

"As soon as possible. Immediately! That's what they all say." The bookseller kept muttering while he clumsily shuffled through a disarrayed pile of folders, papers and leaflets. "I only have one paper ready immediately and that is for the Father here."

The bookseller waved his hand at the anxious prelate. "He is also in dire straits, immediate threat, and now at last we can secure his exit, but that is it!" He slammed one paper atop the others. "Two or three days is as immediate as you'll get. I'm no magician, no, not me—no magician."

"Two or three days is impossible!" Pandora said. "He's to be arrested as a spy tonight and stands no chance to survive. You must do something. Here, take this." She started counting out money onto the pile of papers. "I have all of this to give you, but only for tonight's work. It must be tonight!"

The priest rose from his chair, Pandora's pluck and tender years seeming to have a salutary effect on his frazzled nerves. In his dark cassock, and through the hazy light he seemed to glide rather than walk toward her. Funny, she thought, how in the light she couldn't tell whether this was a priest or a woman, simply clad, without her bonnet. An idea dawned.

"Sir?" She returned to the bookseller, who was checking the money she'd laid out. "Is it difficult to change a paper from an individual to a family?"

"Difficult to change?" the bookman began. "What individual? What family? What do you mean?"

Pandora grabbed the priest's papers and looked them over quickly.

"Here," she said, very annoyed with the dense old man. "Here, where it says family members, where it's blank. Couldn't you put in other names? A wife, a child?"

"Well, yes of course, if there were one, but, Mademoiselle, this is for the priest, there is no family, no wife."

"Fool!" Pandora yelled. "What if there were to be? If we dressed him in a disguise as a woman, no one would know, and you could get three people out at once as a family, without arousing any suspicion whatsoever!"

* * *

"Wait over there, Father," Pandora said pointing to a low pile of crates and trunks stored in the basement. As she bounded up the stairs and rapped the code on the kitchen door, her pride of accomplishment warmed her blood and set her to imagining herself poised on the deck of the great ship that was going to carry her to the shores of England. She began to whistle her own rendition of a sea chantey.

When Peliciàn opened the door Pandora almost fell into the kitchen, as in her fantasy the door had become the ship's rail and she'd leaned too hard on it.

"It's done!" She said thumping the papers onto the table in front of General Miranda. She tried to step back and let him read but her enthusiasm was uncontrollable. "Of course, sir, this is not so simple of a situation," she interrupted. "There are, as you will note, two unexpected turns of the plan, but—"

"Pandora." Miranda said, giving her a rather withering look.

"In these matters the unexpected turns should always be expected." She was pleased with this rather mature thinking but reacting to the general's impatience she went to the basement door and signaled to the priest who was waiting.

"General Miranda!" she pronounced, trying to buoy her self-confidence. "I would like you to meet my mother!"

Peleciàn gasped, General Miranda, rose, papers in hand.

"Come in, Father Ignatius," she said, pulling the timid man up into the kitchen. "Come, come. Don't worry, everyone here is trustworthy."

"Heavens before us!" Peleciàn uttered, blessing herself several times in the deference.

"Bring the poor fellow a chair," Pandora said, feeling her confidence restored.

Completely flustered, Mademoiselle shoved a chair into the back of the frail priest's knees, practically knocking him into the seat before he had time to steady himself.

"What is this all about?" Miranda asked.

"It's quite easy to explain, sir," Pandora said. "Each of us has been confronted with a dilemma. You are in urgent need of papers to secure your exit at once. So it seems is Father Ignatius, and so am I. When I arrived at the bookseller's, he had already made provisions for Father Ignatius, but could not accommodate us as speedily as we needed. I pondered and pondered this difficult problem, and suddenly I seized on this idea. If we were to exit as a family, we could all be placed on the same document without suspicion. When I proposed this to the bookseller and showed him the color of your money, he too found my idea the perfect solution to his and our problem. Within minutes he altered Father Ignatius's paper to read, M. and Mme. Miranda and child—that's me—traveling from Russia through Paris en route to London, granted exit on this day etc., etc."

General Miranda looked closely at the papers in his fist. "It works out quite neatly, don't you think? Father Ignatius has already agreed to disguise himself as my mother, and I of course do not have to change myself as I am a child."

"Yes, thank you. Light is dawning," Miranda said.

"Of course we will have to make Father Ignatius's garb more convincing." She laughed, as did the still rather baffled cleric.

"Most definitely!" Miranda said, a slow grin breaking up his sternness. Then with a crackle of laughter filling the room, he said, "Yes indeed, Pandora, we must adjust his garb."

He has accepted my plan, Pandora thought, a swell of triumph and relief sending her into a little dance.

Only Mademoiselle Peleciàn stood silent and alone near the fire, away from the merry conspirators.

"Nothing good will come of this," she said. "This child is degenerating before my very eyes. She is turning from a common, ill-mannered, ragamuffin into an instrument of sacrilege and blasphemy. General, I must say, with all due respect, you encourage her."

"Mademoiselle?" Father Ignatius said, touching her sleeve. "You must not be so hard on the girl. Remarkably, she has found a solution to several complex problems with a great deal of imagination and aplomb. I must admit to you the prospect of my escape, though necessary, did not put me at ease. I found I am not well suited for treacherous journeys unaccompanied. But, because of the urgency of my plight, I had no choice but to attempt it. I suspect, though, I would somehow have failed, putting far more than my own worthless life in jeopardy. When the girl came and unraveled her charm, I leapt at the notion despite the discomfort of my particular role. She may be impetuous and rough-edged, but her spirit is strong and her deeds full of goodness. No doubt that is a reflection of your pious influence, Mademoiselle."

Pliciàn looked coldly at Father Ignatius, for an uncomfortably long time. Pandora kept her eyes defiantly on the woman.

"Far be it from me not to help a priest. If you will come with me, Father, I will do my best to turn you into a modest woman," she said at last.

"Pandora," General Miranda said, listening for the creak of the stairs as Mademoiselle led the priest aloft. "You have done well as my soldier and followed my orders beyond measure. But you have also been disobedient in your actions regarding my opposition to your leaving France with me, and my clear and adamant intention that you attend the convent school. A truly fine soldier does not disobey any orders, no matter his own want or predilection."

"But, sir," Pandora said. "I did not disobey any of your orders. You did not order me to attend the convent school. You merely said you felt it would be the best thing. I obeyed your order to secure your passage. I was only able to do that under these conditions and so that is what was left for me to do."

"Pandora, I see we can spin this wheel around, and around, and we will not see it the same. Once again I find myself in your debt and with time against us, the papers will be used as stated and we will depart together. But Mademoiselle will take this turn very deep to her soul. She has a stern crust but a soft, warm heart, which has been yours ever since you arrived. Your leaving this way will wound her spirit. Try to make some amends if you can."

***

Pandora stood by the entrance to the tunnel, watching Henri carry the last trunk down the narrow lantern-lit passage to the general at the other end. Father Ignatius followed awkwardly. He was dressed in a slim, black coat with a high collar partially concealing his lower jaw. A tall crowned bonnet was wrapped snug to his cheeks and tied in a large bow under his chin. Pandora shivered, but it wasn't the dampness or cold in the basement that produced her chill; it was the overwhelming excitement and anticipation of the impending journey that made her fingertips and toes feel cold and sent goose pimples across her back.

"Open it, child," said Mademoiselle, who had been standing next to her all this time without saying a word. She extended toward Pandora a small black tin box. Pandora took it out of Mademoiselle's hands and opened it. Folded in a neat circle was Mademoiselle's old rosary, the very one that always hung down from her skirts and announced her imminent presence in any room of the house. In the upper corner, lying on a black velvet ribbon, was a gold locket which Mademoiselle took up and pinched open.

"This is a likeness of St. Anne, Mother of the Virgin Mary, Mother of Mothers. I have loved you, Pandora, as I would love my own. As long as God allows breath to stay in my body, I will be here if you need me. In the meanwhile, I will pray to St. Anne, to watch over you. Now," she bent to Pandora, "kiss me on the cheek and let's make a clean end to it."

With no hesitation Pandora flung herself on Peliciàn's neck and in gasps between sobs she inhaled this woman's smells, the soaps, the fire smoke, the boiling stews, all of which made up her distinct aroma. Mademoiselle held her tight, rocking her ever so slightly back and forth, until there were no more sobs—just silence.

"All right, child." She separated them and adjusted the tear-soaked shoulder of her blouse. "The general is ready. It's time for you to go."

CHAPTER THIRTEEN

Pandora learned early in the voyage from France to England that she was of that breed of creature who belonged on land and not upon the sea. The uncomfortable sensation presented itself almost immediately, as the ship heaved into the rough channel, unfurling her sails to the wind. She was struck so strongly by the undignified malady that it caused her a considerable amount of embarrassment. But her determination to participate fully in every moment of her new adventure was so profound that neither a distorted equilibrium nor the consequences of mal de mer kept her from her objective.

Despite her indisposition she stood on the bow of the ship, shaky legs planted wide apart for security, General Miranda on one side, Father Ignatius on the other, as they sailed up the Thames toward London. Though the river was agitated by a strong north wind, its choppiness seemed almost gentle compared with the roughness of the open sea. This quieted Pandora's stomach even though her color could scarcely be described as rosy. The sun shone crystal clear in the September sky; it was one of those days when the horizon seemed limitless.

When they reached the broad breast of the river, the city of London spread full before them. Just ahead, rising far up above the roofs of all the other buildings was the great round dome of Saint Paul's Cathedral. Pandora heard its deep bell and counted aloud the gongs up to ten o'clock. Then her eye surveyed the shore, moving down the bank until she found what she was looking for. There, exactly like the picture in her book, was the Tower of London—that fortress of doom, so strong and neatly built at the waters edge, its thick stone walls connecting the four towers, each peaked by a deserted flag pole. Pandora closed her eyes and imagined the wives of Henry VIII, waiting in the white tower to be beheaded.

Nearing the London docks, the ship maneuvered carefully among the multitude of others, congesting the harbor from shore to shore, until they finally rested alongside the dock. Then the sails were let down with clamorous speed and they joined the other ships that lay at berth, their masts swaying like a dense forest of denuded trees.

When the gangplank was lowered, Pandora, the general and Father Ignatius stood atop looking out. Everywhere, people feverishly engaged in the transactions of commerce. Peddlers with baskets on their heads hauled everything from flowers to shoelaces.

Fishmongers, holding fresh mackerel, beckoned customers; merchants, tradesmen and passengers, both coming and going, joined with the thwacking of loose halyards against the bare masts in one grand panharmonium.

The intensity of this bustling hive induced in Pandora a feeling of light-headedness, but the moment they disembarked and her feet once again touched solid ground her feeling of relief overtook all. Returning to a stable equilibrium she began to sort and store all that she observed. Standing nearby, a man holding up a hook of fresh mackerel hawked and cajoled every potential customer within reasonable distance.

Pandora listened for familiar words but many were not, and the broken edges of his accent made her wonder if he was speaking English or something entirely different. All around her people moved and maneuvered with a kind of rough enthusiasm, often knocking her off her spot, barely acknowledging their transgressions with a swallowed, "Pr-dn, Miss." It was a feast of sorts to the eyes, ears, nose and spirit. Money changed hands as quickly as an item was chosen, and the carts so overfilled of merchandise made her wonder whether they'd ever be empty. This was not France at all, the pitch was far too strong and the bounty too great.

The general parted the crowd by leading the way to a hackney stand. Pandora swung her old burlap sack securely under her arm, not wanting it to fall prey to some low life working the preoccupied crowd. Anxiously she reached inside and shook the black tin box which held the rosary and locket Mademoiselle Peliciàn had given her. At the hackney stand Miranda negotiated briefly with the drivers of two shiny black coaches. Father Ignatius, having removed his bonnet and wig, lifted Pandora into her carriage.

"Well now, young lady," he said, looking for the first time rather foolish in his "lady's" costume, "I hope we will soon meet again. Though I never thought of it before, my calling indeed is not far removed from that of a mother, and it has been an honor to have pretended to be yours. I am sure God will keep a keen eye on you and remain at your elbow to aid you in your future good deeds, however strange they may be." With a quick kiss on the cheek, he entered his carriage and drove off into the crowded thoroughfare.

Miranda, accompanied by the driver of their carriage, returned to the docked ship to bring back the trunks and Pandora, her queasy stomach now calm but her head full of spectacle and noise, waited and watched.

"Oranges, oranges, fresh Spanish oranges 'ere!"

Standing a few yards away, Pandora saw a little peddler girl. She was approximately the same age as herself, with cherubim shape and the most generous rosy cheeks imaginable. Around her shoulders hung a straw tray laden with oranges. Pandora left the carriage and made her way over to the girl. Stopping just a few feet away, she stared, intently.

"Whatcha lookin' at?" said the child. "Ain't cha ever seen an orange 'afore?"

"Where do you get them?" Pandora asked.

"I get them from Carbonnes," said the girl, pointing toward a long row of warehouses lining one whole side of the piers.

"How much do you make in a day?" Pandora asked.

"Well, that depends on whether it's a good day or a bad one, don't it? Now on a good day I can sell as much as two full trays, but on a bad one, maybe 'alf a tray." She absentmindedly rearranged the top grouping of oranges as she spoke.

"Where do you come from? You speak English funny."

"I am from Paris," Pandora said.

"Oh, is that your father over there?"

They both looked over to the carriage and saw Miranda looking about for Pandora while the driver loaded the trunks.

"No," Pandora said. "I might be looking for work, soon. Do you know of any restaurants around, where they speak French,"

"Nope," the peddler said. "But if you look me up, I could see you gets fixed up proper as a fruit-seller."

"Thank you. I might just do that," Pandora said.

"Ere, 'ave an orange."

Pandora caught the tossed fruit.

"Thanks."

"'Ave a good day. Oranges, oranges, fresh Spanish oranges 'ere." The girl squeezed into the crush of people and disappeared, save for her call. Pandora listened a moment then turned to the general.

He was still wearing the red wig and tinted glasses. He had concocted the disguise to add an extra measure of security to their flight—the green glasses to conceal his visage from any agent who might try to prevent escape, the red wig an artistic touch provided by Pandora.

"Pandora!" Miranda called, seeing her at last.

All during the voyage Pandora had prepared herself for this moment and now that it was at hand she decided to make the first move.

Well, I guess this is the time for our farewell." She extended her hand in as manly a manner as she thought proper.

"I am not sure I understand," Miranda said, not taking her cue nor reaching to shake hands with her.

"Well, sir, I was thinking, since you did not want to bring me in the first place, there is no need for you to feel obliged now that I'm here. I can perfectly well take care of myself. In fact I have already secured myself a good position in the immediate area, so I'm nearly settled already."

When the general removed his glasses, he had the strangest look on his face—one Pandora had never seen. It was halfway between a twinkling eye and a great burst of laughter restrained. Unnerved, she prattled on.

"If at any time you find you need me, you can inquire at Carbonnes." She pointed to the warehouses. "They'll know my whereabouts."

"Pandora, do you think after your bold and successful solution to our escape and your determined resolve to accompany me to London, that I would now have you go off by yourself? Or that I would not want you to accompany me to my home and family here?"

"I don't know, sir. I may be in the way as I was be—"

Pandora stopped short of letting him know what had bothered her in Paris. She wasn't sure it wouldn't be true here as well.

"Be in the way? What kind of foolishness are you talking? But if you find my home does not suit you well, then you may leave without obligation. In any case, why don't you at the very least, come and have a good meal and a sound night's rest? After a rough journey, all soldiers need rest and a good repast. Tomorrow, you can depart if you still wish."

"Yes, I suppose I could do that."

"It's settled then." Miranda lifted her into the carriage with a hasty move and tapped the driver to get under way.

As soon as they left the proximity of the docks and were slowly winding their way along the narrow back streets to the main thoroughfare, Miranda removed his wig and settled back in his seat. Turning onto Fleet Street, Pandora felt the carriage pick up pace, and she leaned forward to look out at the sights going by. When they passed the facade of St. Paul's at Ludgate, Miranda began to point out other landmarks and explain their histories and architecture.

Pandora only half listened. She was observing the vast differences between the Paris streets and those of London. There were no roving bands of "citoyens", crying for blood. The bake shops had no endless lines of angry women futilely hoping for a morsel to bring home. Why, even the peddler girl on the wharf had rosy cheeks and a healthy demeanor. At every turn there was another view of this lively and industrious city.

Yet Pandora was not optimistic about life at the general's home. She knew little of his English life, and she feared Sarah Andrews. The mother of his son was no Mademoiselle Peliciàn and would not open her heart and home to an intruding orphan from a foreign land. Pandora was glad she'd already made productive inquiries, just in case.

Her sudden sullenness so weighted the air in the hackney that the general could not help but notice it.

"Are you still under the influence of the rough seas? Or are the sights of this great city of no interest to you?"

"Neither!" Pandora said, making sure her flat tone conveyed her desire to be left alone.

With a jolt the carriage turned sharply. A sign read Dover Street, then Pandora saw they'd turned off onto a street named Grafton. Miranda buttoned the top of his jacket as the carriage swayed from side to side.

"We're here," Miranda said, just as the driver pulled up the horses. Pandora looked at the house. She saw a high stone wall with the branches of two staid sycamores extending well over the top of it. A door with the number 27 was carved in the center of this wall, and when Pandora alighted she saw that Grafton Street was only two blocks in length and that clearly the houses had the style of the energetic well-to-do. Her apprehension was growing.

Inside the courtyard the abundant leaves on the trees produced a cool shade. The house itself was very broad and had three stories, the third peaking into two sloping facades, each with small paned windows just under the eaves. The home was made entirely of brick, weathered into many variegations. On either side there was a four-spouted chimney. Each floor had identical windows, and the main door was solid oak, with five steps leading from it.

On a ladder raised to the second story stood an immense man washing the windows and singing in the most horrible voice imaginable. He looked like a giant misplaced from some fairy tale. His head was so large it demanded two sets of shoulders, though his were certainly ample. The hands which were busy rubbing glass in time to his horrid tune dwarfed both bucket and rag.

The general snuck up to the ladder and, with full military bearing, shouted, "Topham!" The ladder trembled from the giant's start. But when he saw who it was addressing him, he bounded down with a broad grin that exposed an overstocked mouth of multi-shaded teeth. He grabbed the general full around the shoulders, and proceeded to dance a wild, interpretive jig.

"'Eese 'ere! 'Eese 'ere!" the man called Topham shrieked.

Suddenly the front door burst open, and Pandora watched a collection of jubilant people issue forth, all talking at once in the most impassioned manner. In their eagerness to greet the general, they formed a tight knot around him, leaving Pandora at liberty. She noticed that in their enthusiasm no one had closed the front door of the house. Her curiosity far too stimulated to wait for them to notice her and bring her into the claque, she approached the house on her own and stepped inside.

There was a wide stream of sunlight emanating from an open door off to the left side of the foyer. A large stairway rose on the right wall and turned in a graceful sweep into a balcony above. Pandora could see the shine of a large oval mirror that hung mid-wall on this balcony. Before her the room narrowed to a long corridor, which made a dead end at a large ornate door some distance away. The entrance hall itself had a huge brass chandelier hanging in the center, with many curved arms all of which came from what appeared to be the mouths of lions. The candles came out of tulip-shaped holders with flame carvings, and the whole thing hung from the middle of a gold leafed circle molded to the ceiling. The walls were covered in a shiny cloth with a floral pattern. There were many paintings which were hard to see clearly in the dim light. Against the stairwell was a long table with a huge urn full of flowers. A giant round rug covered the floor, its center black, then ringed with flowers of burgundy, rose, violet and green. Pandora started toward the light.

"You must be Pandora." A voice startled her, she looked behind her, then up the stair. Then she saw two feet sticking out the door of the lit room.

"Hello," she said, and waited for the feet to move. "Yes, I am," she said. "Who are you?" She continued to wait, expectantly.

Finally, a figure emerged. He was rather tall, but totally ill-proportioned. His feet were far too long for the thin ankles which rose up out of them into legs that seemed to end way above the normal waist line. The arms, also thin, hung limply at his sides. Long-fingered hands passed below his knees. He had broad shoulders, a good neck and an angular face, and there was promise of handsomeness in the sculpted cheeks, strong chin and black hair. Pandora saw the unquestionable mark of General Miranda, in the boy's dark complexion.

"You must be Leander," she said, causing the boy to wiggle his fingers nervously and drop his head in an awkward bow. She had an inclination to giggle at his bashfulness, but knew better, although the idea to tickle him accompanied her musing. He was, despite his timidity, a comely lad.

"Are you going to be staying here?" Leander asked.

"I don't know," Pandora said. "I don't think I will be staying but I did promise the general I would come for dinner anyway. Why aren't you outside with the rest of them? Don't you want to greet your father?"

"I will wait for the hubbub to die down." His face flushed a bit. He pushed his hair off his forehead.

"I am not very good at crowds," he said.

"Oh. Well, what are you very good at?"

Leander smiled in a way that made her think he liked her. "I don't know the answer to that, really. My tutor, Mr. Barry, says I am quite passable at my studies. And I like adventures very much." He looked straight at her now.

"What kind of adventures?"

"The dangerous kind."

"Leander!" A voice from the doorway interrupted, preventing Pandora from getting down to the heart of Leander's revelation.

"That's my mother. She's come to drag me out."

Sarah stood framed in the door. The others were peering from behind her with unrestrained curiosity.

"You must be the remarkable Pandora," she said, extending her a hand, a musical lilt giving her words a singsong quality. "I am Sarah."

Pandora took her hand. It was slender but very firm in grip and warm to the touch. She was wearing a decolleté black lace blouse, which exposed the milk white skin of her neck and bosom. Her skirt was green and white striped, a sort of shiny material that shimmered more so because of the gold threads woven in and out of the stripes.

"Come along." Sarah put her arm around Pandora's shoulders, then sternly summoned Leander to follow her down the stairs, back to the courtyard where General Miranda was trying to guide the household into a rag-tag line. There was so much conversation going on amongst the others he finally gave up and turned to the two children. Seeing Leander, he embraced him across the shoulders with his long arms and beamed proudly.

"How are you, son?" he said to Leander, pulling him in tighter.

"Just fine, Father, sir. How are you?"

Pandora saw that Leander's color had become quite crimson and that his stiff body and formal tone conveyed how really uncomfortable he was as the center of attention. The entire household also seemed aware of this. They stopped yammering and were all watching and waiting for a further exchange between father and son. A concerned awkwardness hung like a mist in the air.

"You've grown a good deal. I hardly would recognize you," Miranda said. "I left a boy and have returned to find a young man," he concluded, with a good bit of gusto that provoked a hearty laugh from all save Leander. His mortification only deepened at the collective attempt to put him at ease. Miranda was undaunted.

"I see you have already met Pandora so there is no need to introduce you. But now let's have her meet the others. Ladies and gentlemen!" He pulled Pandora forward. "I want to introduce you all to the most exceptional young lady. One to whom I owe a debt so great I fear I shall never repay it."

Before Pandora could curtsey or mutter a greeting, she found herself standing face to face with the first person in the line.

"This fine gentleman," Miranda began, "of positively pantegruelesque proportions, is Mr. Topham—who, according to my reckoning, is the strongest fellow of whom these British Isles may boast." Everyone laughed and applauded this assertion.

"But his strength, formidable as it is, is surpassed only by his kindness and loyalty."

Topham looked skyward and grinned self-consciously. Then he tossed Pandora a broad wink, to which she rendered a dainty curtsey. The giant man bellowed with glee at such a fine gesture. Pandora thought even Mademoiselle Peliciàn would have been proud of her delicate execution.

"This is Carmen Mendoza and her daughter Rosa," Miranda said, ushering Pandora down the line. She hesitated in front of

Carmen, who cupped her face between her warm, chubby hands and kissed her wetly on both cheeks. The woman called Carmen declared with unbridled fervor some no doubt endearing phrase in her native Portuguese. Her oversized bosom and square figure made her stature appear even more squat than it really was. Pandora immediately sensed the maternal blood which coursed through her. Beside her was her daughter Rosa, a salacious beauty with jet-black, waist-length hair, taut, olive skin and the promise of merriment in her light-green eyes. But Pandora barely took notice, because next to her stood the strangest looking fellow she'd ever seen.

"James Barry," Miranda said.

He was short of rough-hewn build, yet when she looked at his hands she saw they were delicate. His face was pockmarked, his gray wig stringy and wild, but his peculiarity came more from a force that emanated from within him. Its intensity was at least as great as General Miranda's.

"Historical painter of the Royal Academy," Miranda announced. "Friend of the highest order—and teacher of everyone he meets! If you decide to stay," Miranda said aside to Pandora, "Your education will be in his most capable hands."

"Yes," Barry said, picking up the thread. "And I'll have you know right now I am a stern taskmaster. It is my belief that one must pay a price to learn. True learning has great cost and even greater responsibility. To see things as they really are brings about a strong discomfort."

Though he addressed his remarks to Pandora, his volume made him accessible to all, as if he were on stage.

"I'll give you an example of which I speak. It will make my point of view clear. You are an orphan?" he said. "You have undoubtedly considered this a great misgiving. From one point of view, call it the emotional one, this is true. But from an equally valid perception one could consider it a great advantage."

"Whatever do you mean, sir?" Pandora heard herself ask. He laughed a laugh full of snorts and guffaws.

"It's quite simple, quite obvious. When one has no past, no personal tradition, one is unencumbered from the normal restraints such as familial expectations, the confines of religion or the narrowness of class—all are things which impede real thought and bold action and prevent most people from attaining greatness."

"I never thought of it that way before," Pandora said.

"Ah, but that is why one needs a teacher; to make the unseen visible."

"I suppose so."

"Ladies and gentlemen," Sarah said, closing the moment with impeccable timing. "Unless the French have robbed the general of his taste for food, he must be starved. Let us retire to the table." With incomparable flourish, she lifted her skirts and preceded her brood into the house.

The loquacious group spent the afternoon in the kitchen, Pandora sitting in the center of a bench, one of a pair gracing either side of the long table. They dined on cold mutton, salted cod and Carmen's deliciously smooth yellow flan. All during the meal Pandora watched Leander stare at her but each time she faced him with a smile, he returned to his plate where he busied himself arranging and rearranging his food, never once eating a morsel.

When Rosa began clearing away the dishes Pandora found herself in a quandary. She did not know whether she was expected to assist, as she'd always done with Mademoiselle. But since no one motioned to her to do so—and she'd only agreed to be a guest for the evening—she decided to exercise her privilege and remain seated.

Topham rose to stoke the fire and rekindle the flames.

"Well, General," he said. "Your letters have been grand, but they're a poor substitute for one of your tales."

Everyone chorused agreement, and as the general eased into his soldier's story, Pandora saw Leander come alive. Rosa joined her mother at the end of the bench and leaned against her. Sarah, who was already sitting on the general's right, picked up her Turkish macrame and began knotting. James Barry, at the end of the table, gingerly cut the peel from an apple and sliced it in quarters. Pandora imagined that this was how it must always be whenever the general was home. Then she turned all her attention again to Leander, whose face was growing luminous with enchantment. She watched him watch his father. She could see that this shy boy was most comfortable with matters of the imagination and that despite himself he loved his father dearly.

The candles melted down, the light dimmed, and the kitchen took on the magic of a theater, with the general its sole actor. With a fluid gesture, practiced poise and precisely placed inflection in his every phrase, he carried his audience back to France and the revolution. He told of a glorious dream turned into a nightmare—of tyrants and heroes and the damnable guillotine. He shocked them with the tale of Bicetre and the "Iron Maiden" that could lop off ten heads at once.

"Imagine," he said. "An entire society gone mad. A lunatic asylum run by the most deranged of the inmates. Paris, the most beautiful city in the world, Pandemonium—the capitol of Hell, presided over by the devil himself—Maximilien Robespierre. There is one at this table who with her very own eyes witnessed the execution of the dragon and brought to my prison cell such a vivid description of the historical event that I and my fellows felt we too had been there."

Pandora, eager for the opportunity to shine in Leander's eyes, began without hesitation to tell her tale.

CHAPTER FOURTEEN

Rosa poured the thick rich coffee into each of the small cups she brought from the pantry. The aromatic smell certainly tempted Pandora to keep her eyes open just a little longer to savor it and the colorful, creamy trifle sitting before Sarah waiting to be spooned around. But the long journey and its eventful conclusion weighed far too heavily on her and she began to fade. Her head dropped to her chest, then jerked up as she tried futilely to stay with the wafting conversation surrounding her. She felt Sarah touch her arm, then her hand cup her head and draw it to her shoulder.

"Look," Barry interrupted the general's point.

"She's gone to sleep."

There was a pause. Everyone smiled benevolently at Pandora, her own expression angelically becalmed by quiet repose. Her springy red curls were still, but fell in merry disarray about her face.

"She came among us," the general began, his whisper full and rich. "She lived under a bridge. She had neither mother, nor father—not even a name. Magically, she appeared during the darkest of days—a ragged little courier of soaps and messages. Very soon I anticipated her visits as one does events of tantamount importance and, though life was black, she managed to worm her way into my despondent heart. Then once she knew I was hers, like any other woman she started making demands. She wanted to learn—to be taught how to read, how to write, how to make sense of numbers—and we all were only too eager to acquiesce. Our lives once again had purpose. Never had a 'faculty' a more able and willing pupil. And whenever the guillotine called one of us away – another rose to take his place."

Topham's eyes began to water, Sarah pressed the child closer. The room was very still.

"I do not know how I would have endured those days without her. For I had forgotten that it is not the present that really matters but the future. This child is blessed with a tenacity for life that I have never seen equaled on any field of battle."

As if sensing all the good feeling and attention radiating towards her, Pandora opened her eyes. For an instant she couldn't remember where she was, but when she saw all eyes on her, she sat up and looked at them one by one. She stopped in surprise at Mr. Topham, whose big face was soaked with tears, his shoulders drooping forward. What could she have missed? General Miranda must have had some sad tale to tell to evoke such a response from the giant.

"Pandora…." Sarah nudged her gently. "My sweet darling, I think it's time for you to go to bed."

Pandora was grateful for the promise of soft pillows and warm covers and obediently followed Sarah's lead, standing next to her while she lit a lamp.

"Please, mother," Leander sprang up from his place. "May I show our guest to her room?"

"Yes, of course." Sarah smiled, handing him the lamp. "But don't keep the poor, exhausted girl up with any prattle. She's a very tired young lady, and tomorrow is another day."

"Good night and thank you," Pandora said to all.

"Good night, dear child. Sleep well, pleasant dreams," she heard them say, as Leander drew her away.

Though her exhaustion had overpowered her, as soon as they got into the cool hallway and began passing from one room to another, she was rejuvenated and could not help but notice that each room was adorned with wonderful and beautiful things. They reached the loggia, and Pandora listened to the pleasant tapping her and Leander's shoes made as they seemed to glide across the mirror-polished marble floor.

She gazed up at the octagonal shapes in the ceiling, one inside the other. The wall opposite the windows was covered top to bottom with paintings of enormous size and epic themes. She wanted to stop and get a full view but Leander pressed on to the end of the broad open stretch, until they reached a door that appeared to be twice as tall as all the rest. Leander passed her the lamp, and she glimpsed at her own reflection in its highly polished rosewood veneer.

Leander heaved open the heavy portal and when Pandora stepped inside she found herself standing in a huge library two stories high, double tiered. Quickly, she went to the center of the room and lifted the lamp as high as she could to see all around this amazing place. A railed balcony ringed the entire second level. At the far end stood a black marble fireplace with Doric columns. An oval skylight graced the dome ceiling and cast down a hazy circle of light onto the long wooden table below, and everywhere, all around, packed tight together, up to the ceiling, were shelves full of books.

"Incroyable," she said.

"Come," Leander said, preceding her up a circular stair. They walked along the balcony, stopping at an open door set inside the bookcases. The window inside the room was partially opened, its panes shiny from the mist. A small bed full of lacy and printed pillows trimmed one wall; in the corner a fat, overstuffed chair with matching ottoman was set. A writing desk faced out the window and opposite the desk was a wooden dresser with a yellow wash basin and matching pitcher atop.

"This used to be the general's reading room," Leander said.

"But Sarah thought, judging from what the general said about you in his letters, that it would be the ideal room for you."

Stunned and now wide awake, Pandora sat on the little bed. Even part of one wall in this little room had a bookcase full of volumes.

"Do you have any *Cooke's Travels?*" she asked, trying to see what might be in her shelves.

"We have many travel books; we have a whole travel section." Leander grabbed the lamp. He called back, "We have *Magellan's Travels, Cortez and the Incas,*" as he ran out, leaving Pandora in the dark. "I'll bring them to you...."

In no time he returned, loaded down with books, with the lantern precariously balanced on top.

Pandora jumped up. "You'll set a fire." She laughed, grabbing the lantern and several of the top volumes. Leander laid out the rest.

"This one's my favorite, the drawings are so inviting." He opened a large brown book as Pandora sat on one side and he on the other. The night grew deeper while the two turned page after page, Leander explaining his love of this or that, Pandora's eyes sparkling at the bounty and his intimate knowledge of each.

Sarah came up as the rose of morning was crawling across the flowered rug of the little room. When she peeked in, she saw both of the children stretched across the bed, their heads buried in the mountain of pillows, books were open everywhere, on the floor, on the chair, the bed and the chest. She went in, closed the window and threw a crocheted coverlet over Pandora.

"Leander," she coaxed her groggy son,"come along." She put her arm around him and led him to the doorway.

Through his sleep blurred eyes, he turned for one last look at his new friend.

CHAPTER FIFTEEN

Topham sat atop the carriage, his huge head hidden under his broad-brimmed hat. The bright red scarf, which was draped like an ox's yoke round his neck, made him more clown-like than ever. Pandora watched him through the window, his powerful shoulders and arms maneuvering the horse along the narrow back streets until they came out onto the great Surry Road. She watched him doff his hat toward everyone he knew with the sort of grand gesture generally employed by those seeking high office. She had already grown so fond of this gentle man that she found everything he did both entertaining and endearing.

As they neared the Egyptian Obelisk, which stood incongruously at the bottom of the road, Topham turned around and saw the child looking up at him. "My, my, ain't you the lucky one. Your second day in London and already a trip to the Royal Circus.

Topham pulled their carriage in behind another, and the horse walked without his guidance, as they inched their way toward the dense crowd under the marquee of the theater.

"I promise," Topham said, leaning closer to the window filling the view with his merry face, "You'll see things tonight that will cause you to doubt the truth of your own eyes. It's spectacular, marvelous, formidable in the utmost!"

Earlier in the day Pandora and Sarah had gone to buy her a new dress. She had never before worn such an elegant garment. The softly gathered long skirt was a bit difficult to walk in and the high collar of her cape made her sit stiffly in the carriage, but it was all right because she saw that Sarah, sitting across from her, was also very straight in her elegant clothes. It surely was the correct thing to do. Sarah had powdered her face to a porcelain white but her lips and cheeks shone a soft pink from a gloss she had applied. Pandora couldn't stop looking at her beautiful face, framed all around by the fold of her bonnet. Her beauty and the strong scent of the rose perfume she wore dominated the atmosphere inside the carriage. When she was grown she hoped she too would have the ease and elegance that Sarah had. But for now her excitement made her hands perspire. So she kept them at her sides, fearing she would leave wet marks on the lap of her dress before she even got inside the theater.

"He's not exaggerating, you know," Leander said, leaning across. "Wait until you see the ballet and pantomime. I guarantee you there is nothing like it in the world and certainly there is nothing like it in Paris."

Pandora started to mount a defense of her birthplace, but her desire not to antagonize or offend any of them stopped her. She managed instead a little smile.

"It's already six-o'clock, General," Topham hollered. "I'm afraid this is as close as we're going to get." Climbing down, he tipped his hat and smiled broadly at two young Irish nannies. They giggled and took each other's arms as they hurried away in the direction of the theater.

"That's fine, Topham. We can manage very well from here," the general said, stepping out and helping Sarah alight, with his special Latin grace. Leander helped Pandora with an awkward imitation of his father. When she alighted she gently smoothed her skirt.

"What are you thinking?" Leander asked, while they pressed ahead, barely keeping Sarah and the general in sight.

"Nothing!"

"Well, aren't you impressed? Don't you think this is grand, all these people? Are you happy to be here? Aren't you excited we are going to the circus?"

"It's very nice," she said, trying to be polite, but she wanted to see the sights without interruption, which, given the compressing crowd as they neared the entrance to the circus, was difficult enough for her without Leander's questions.

When at last they had swept into the theater with the rest of the mob, Pandora was truly taken by what she saw. Overhead, the domed ceiling hovered like the sky. It was painted with flying cherubs, surrounded by white, puffy clouds. Underneath was a great sweeping circle of green and gold balconies, strung together with painted ribbons which seemed to catch the crystal sconces in their bows. Right down in front of the stage was a riding ring, manicured without a flaw, and everywhere people were dressed in the finest fashion. The patois of greetings and laughter was accompanied by the musicians warming their instruments. Pandora watched a huge man sitting with his tuba, engaged in animated conversation with a tiny fellow, standing behind two kettle drums and a collection of bells and cymbals. She would never admit it to Leander, but things looked very promising indeed.

After they were seated in their box, Pandora leaned over the front, savoring every vision, while Leander kept up a nonstop explanation of each new development. The air was filled with the mingling smells of horses, perfume, and smoked chestnuts and wet with anticipation. Then the kettle drums began to roll and a hopeful silence swept the hall.

Into the center ring came a rider, ramrod straight, aboard a prancing buttermilk Lipizzan. Up the horse went on its hind legs, pawing the air and turning in a tight circle, while it's master broadly waved his hat, in acceptance of the warm welcome of the crowd. Now that the evening's entertainment was about to be served, they clapped vigorously.

"Welcome, welcome! Ladies and gentlemen and British citizens from all corners of His Majesty's Realm. The Royal Circus is warmed by your presence and inspired to present an evening that will not only thrill and excite you, but will certainly lure your souls to fly to the loftiest of heights. So without further ado, I, your humble servant, Mr. Hughes, riding master of this daring troupe, call the finest equestrians in all the world to let the entertainment begin."

At that moment, Mr. Hughes's great white steed reared up again and performed a quick pirouette before cantering out on the audience's applause. Pandora studied Leander while this master horseman performed. She applauded when he did and laughed when he laughed; she followed his cue. But, when the band struck the fanfare, heralding the arrival of the first rider, she no longer needed to follow her mentor.

The event itself took charge. Three horses came galloping into the ring, mounted by a man clad in black boots, white britches and blue jacket trimmed with dazzling gold buttons and fringed epaulets. He straddled all three animals, holding their reins in one hand, while saluting the enthusiastic crowd with the other. After one successful manége around the ring, another horseman galloped in from the other side of the arena. He rose up with one leg in the saddle of his coal black gelding, the other jauntily placed between the horse's ears; all the while he blew a charge through a long brass trumpet.

Then, while the tempo of the band increased, in charged a piebald colt carrying a man in full headstand. He was balanced atop two buckets which rested on the saddle. He held his reins in the right hand and in the left a bouquet of silk flowers. Above him, his legs were crossed as if he were in easy recline. Dropping their reserve, the crowd oohed, ahhed, whistled and stomped, but Pandora was motionless with admiration, frozen mid-clap.

Next there appeared a beautiful lady, on tiptoe who wove breathtakingly close in and out of the other cantering steeds. She wore a long, fur-lined gown covered with glass beads that glittered and shimmered in a dazzling rainbow light. She broke the air with the crackle of her long, black whip as she guided her animal with one hand. When the woman's horse reared and bolted, she never once lost her position. Pandora joined the ovation. The band played a military march, not well, but with such gusto that at one point the entire audience kept time with the energetic music makers.

When the horses and riders finally left the ring, Pandora sat down, her eyes wide, her face flushed.

She looked over toward Leander who sat with an "I told you so!" expression on his face. Then the great red curtain across the stage parted, revealing a painted backdrop of blooming heather climbing over a rocky hillside. The rest of the stage was transformed into the Scottish highlands. When the curtain had completely disappeared, three bagpipers arrived in full Scots costume. As they stopped in the uppermost corner of the stage and began to play their pipes, two dancers leapt out from the wings on either side.

"That's Mr. and Mrs. Byrne," Leander whispered, with a tremor of excitement. "He's ours, but she is from Italy—Rossi was her name."

As the pipers played a baleful tune, the couple danced, he leaping and turning, she flitting hither and yon until they came together in a duet which revealed their undying love for one another.

Bored with this artificial spectacle of feigned and overdone emotions, Pandora turned her attention to Leander, whose reaction was quite the opposite. Curiously, he seemed more fascinated and absorbed in this enactment than he had in the exciting equestrian feats and as she looked at him she saw he was subtly moving to the music and quietly humming its tune. She imagined how he would look as a grown man, his sharply chiseled features filling out and molding into a strong swarthy visage. His dark eyes would lose their self-consciousness and become calm and more set. His scrawny neck would thicken just right to support his regal Spanish head and his gangly arms and legs. She could see him becoming muscular and powerful.

The band reached a crescendo. Mr. Byrne lifted his wife up into the air, suspending her over his head. Her gossamer skirts flowed behind her, her face caught in the light, sincerely expressing a serene sense of love and pleasure. Pandora felt a strange pull in her chest. Leander's rapt face, his thick black mane of hair kept her attention all through the polite applause of the audience.

When the Egyptian pantomime began, she returned to her fantasy of the future. She saw herself with Leander near a huge fireplace in their own library, reading stories aloud. The swell of exotic music fanned her imagination and made her daydreams almost palpable.

When they left the theater her head was in a whirl. She wanted very much for Leander to take hold of her hand. By the time they were settled in their carriage again, heading home, everything about this day and place was perfectly wonderful—the fog which closed them in, the clatter of the wheels on the cobbles which set the steady homeward rhythm. Even Topham's dissonant singing enhanced her sense of well-being.

"Well, Pandora," Miranda said, taking her attention away from her secret thoughts. "What do you think of our England,"

"Oh," she said, "I think it is just fine, sir—ever so fine."

In the darkened carriage she let her eyes return and remain unselfconsciously on the boy across from her.

CHAPTER SIXTEEN

"Tragedy, my children, is decreed by God, and once the die is cast, nothing in the power of man can be done to avert it." Nearly two years later James Barry, the hard-featured, pock-pitted Irishman was under full sail, and as the winter winds rattled the oval skylight of the library, the teacher marched up and down along the edge of the great claw-footed table, sawing the air with his incongruously delicate hands.

"The fate of Romeo and Juliet was sealed irrevocably by their uncontrollable passions. But even if they had chosen to deny their love, where would it have led them," he asked, leaning across the table toward Leander and Pandora. "To what noble purpose? To what glorious end? All anyone who chooses a life without passion can hope to achieve is emptiness. And sadly, my children, this is the preferred choice of most."

Barry paused. A hush fell over the library with the power of the point.

"But don't despair, there are those who save our feeble race from complete ignominy, those few rare individuals whose souls have been kindled by the spark of courage, who follow their passions wherever they may lead. These are our heroes. Sometimes their lives are tragic, sometimes they are not, but they are always glorious!"

"God rest ye merry, gentlemen, let nothing you dismay." From a distance away, came the awful sound of Topham's singing. Pandora and Leander looked at each other with amusement. Until now, the two students and their teacher had not been aware of anything other than their lessons, not even the fast fading daylight, which came so quickly these December days. But Topham's caroling would not be ignored and as it grew nearer, all three of them turned their attention toward the door.

"Remember, Christ our Savior was born on Christmas day!" At last Topham arrived in the room and James Barry's hard stare brought his warbling to an immediate end. The two large logs he brought for the fire were lying across his muscular arms, and his head and shoulders were soaked with rain.

"Sorry for the interruption, Professor," he said. "Thought you could do with a little more warmth in here." He dropped the logs in front of the fireplace and shook his head like a big shaggy dog, the flying water sizzling as it hit the bed of glowing embers. "And while I'm here, I'll light the lamp. You don't want these poor children to go blind do you, Mr. Barry?"

"My dear Mr. Topham," Barry began, with tongue-in-cheek sternness, "I'll have you know you just interrupted a crucial lesson on the nature of tragedy." Moving to Topham while he spoke, Barry puffed himself up in a playful way, but since he was a smallish man, just under middle size, no amount of posturing could make him appear anything but diminutive next to the giant.

"Begging your pardon," Topham said, joining the game, while he threw the logs on the fire as if they were twigs. "The real tragedy would be to work these poor little wretches right through Christmas Eve without even a taste of Carmen's fine plum pudding."

Pandora and Leander started to laugh at their two favorite characters, whose disparate figures were perfectly set off by the rejuvenated fire. Pandora's face had become accentuated by a strong chin which seemed to be growing somewhat ahead of her other features, and a slight bosom bloomed under her smock. Leander had lost most of his physical awkwardness in the past two years and was an even more handsome young man, very tall, with a distinctive carriage, though his shy eyes remained tentative and soft.

"Mr. Topham," Barry said, "you may do us the great service of illuminating the room and thus expedite my task of continuing with Mr. Shakespeare a bit longer. Then we will celebrate this most remarkable birth by devouring Carmen's superb goose with the rest of you." He went back to the long table, which was covered from end to end with the books and papers used in the education of his two pupils. "A curious thing," he continued to himself, "why all of Christendom stops on this day to celebrate the birth of a poor Jewish boy, born in a stable eighteen hundred and two years ago. Perhaps it is a miracle indeed."

"You know Mr. Barry, sir," Topham said, winking at the children from behind their teacher's back, "You're a fine fellow, but I never understand a word you say."

"Nevertheless," said Barry, his voice trailing off as he stared nowhere in particular, "It's a curious thing."

***

"Come all ye ladies and gents," boomed a voice from across the dimly lit room. "I am Father Christmas and I have come to bring you cheer!" Topham's costume achieved the penultimate, his towering height was increased by a high stovepipe hat, wreathed with a circle of red-berried holly. His features were obscured with a carrot nose, which was tied to his ears. In place of hair, he sported tufts of pine branches interspersed with more red and white berries, and his massive frame was covered in a cloak fashioned from fresh ivy, cascading all the way to the floor, jauntily fastened at the throat with a bright red ribbon.

"Now," he began, "I will feed the fire this yule log. If it bursts into flame and burns through and through a good year will be had, by all of you."

Topham picked up a large gnarled root and heaved it onto the fire, sending a spray of glittering sparks racing up the chimney. "Bring forth," he called, "the illumination of good will for the coming year!"

Smoke began to surround the log, little blue flames kissed it and the popping of lesser logs filled the silence as Sarah and the general, presiding at the head of the well-stocked table, waited with all the other celebrants in dignified anticipation for the fire to herald in the holiday festivities.

Using a long pine twig as a taper, which he pulled from beneath his hat, Topham lit two fat ornately carved Christmas candles which sat atop the highboy. From down the hall, the steady beat of a tin drum could be heard, soon followed by the voices of children singing,

"Now Christmas is come,
Let us beat up our drum
And bring all our neighbors together!"

The first one to enter the room was the neighbor boy Christophoro, the honorable drum major of this little parade. Upon seeing the dozen or so elegantly dressed members of his audience, he began to assault his drum with exaggerated vigor and grand style. His impish face was completely covered by blackened cork, and his blond head was crowned with a bower of threaded nuts, currants, and berries. A brown Chatelet adorned his long liver-colored coat, under which he clomped in two grown-up sized galoshes, making a sham of his proud entrance.

"Mr. Mince Pie has arrived," Topham announced, "and his presence is greatly essential!"

Christophoro's parents smiled proudly to each other and Sarah nodded with fond approval of their boy's accomplishment. Then, while he marched madly about, Topham summoned the next pageanteer. "The fair Maid Marian she be. Come hither and tell us what thou dost see!" Pandora came through the doorway at an even gait, her voice a little strident, her pitch not quite true. Nonetheless, she sang with assertive confidence.

"When the neighbors appear,
Let us make them good cheer,
so that they pay no heed,
to the weather!"

Her lush velvet dress was strategically gathered and tied with red and green bows, each holding small sprigs of mistletoe. Sarah had applied a blush of rouge to her cheeks, and as she marched she managed to balance, with utmost elegance, the high conical hat from which fell a long trailing white veil. Everyone in the room applauded her charm and beauty, while in the doorway Carmen and Rosa, who had created these costumes could be seen beaming with delight.

"And where, Lady Marian, is your noble Robin Hood," asked Topham. Everyone started to talk and look toward the doorway, but the entrance remained empty, and all that could be heard were

Carmen's stern whispers coming from the hail. Finally Leander appeared, his face aglow with mortification. He had on a leaf green cap, graced with a long pheasant feather. His legs were dressed in chocolate brown tights, and his deerskin tunic was cinched with a black belt. He barely managed to make his verse audible as he took his place next to the others.

"For in here it is warm
and we are out of the storm,
so say us all together!"

With a flourish Christophoro ended his drumming, and the black of his face split into a gap-toothed grin. Those seated around the table stood and cheered, "MERRY CHRISTMAS!" Then General Miranda rose, a small crystal glass in hand, and proposed the toast. "I lift my glass to honor this fine and exceptional gathering, I pray the yule log will burn all through the night, and thus bring luck and goodness into this home. MERRY CHRISTMAS!"

"Merry Christmas!" They all shouted again, and stood raising their glasses towards each other and over the evergreen centerpiece on the table. Carmen, who had already had too much to drink during the preparation of the banquet, was so swept up in the felicity of the moment that she brushed a few sentimental tears from her shiny red face, and began to sing in a light contralto voice:

"Joy to the world,
the Lord has come,
Let Earth receive her King..."

"Look over there, yours is the long thin one on the bottom," Pandora whispered to Leander, her attention still on the gaily wrapped boxes stacked on the highboy. When she turned to catch his expression, the reluctant Robin Hood was nowhere to be found. That miserable little bastard, she thought, precious little Leander has to do something he doesn't want to do and now he's gone off to sulk. Forcing everyone to wonder about him. Well not me, I'll drag that temperamental little ass back here with tongs in his nose if need be!"

While a stream of newly arrived guests were being greeted by the general, Pandora unobtrusively backed out of the room.

Once in the clear, she made haste. Grabbing hold of her conical hat, she ran down the hall toward the library. "Poor Prince Leander has fled to his castle," she fumed, and despite the obstacle of her over-long skirts which kept catching her feet, her ire forced a furious, if awkward, pace. "What a selfish little brick-brained brat he is! I just can't stand him!" she muttered, as she neared her destination. Bursting through the doors, she found Leander just where she knew he would be, sitting on the floor of the balcony, his green hat by his side. "Oh no, Leander," she shouted, as she stormed up the stairs obstinate skirts lifted. "Banish it from your mind altogether, it's Christmas Eve and you're not going to hide in here all night. You're not a bloody tortoise!"

"I know perfectly well who and what I am and I do not need some Parisian street rat to tell me!"

"I may be beneath your noble class, my lord, but at least I am capable of considering others. Which is an ability you seem to lack."

"Oh please!" Leander said opening his book, creating a screen between them.

"Now you listen to me, Leander," she said, snatching it away. "The rest of the guests are all arriving. You must come this very instant!"

"Not on your life, Miss Holy Sanctimony," he said, bolting to his feet. "I've had quite enough Christmas, thank you. Now just go back to the party in your ridiculous costume and leave me be!"

"What is the matter with you? Why are you in such a state? It's a lovely party."

"What's the matter with me, you ask? Pandora, you are a bigger dummy than I ever imagined! Just look at me, look at how they dress me! Like some medieval fool! And if that weren't insult enough, I am commanded to recite in front of everyone a silly rhyme which makes no sense whatsoever. Why, I thought I would expire right there on the spot."

"There you go again," she said, cutting him off, "chained like a dog to your stunted little fancies. You know what's the matter with you Leander? You're just a coward."

"And you, of course, never feel the least bit afraid?"

"No, not at all," Pandora replied, with a sweet smile and charming giggle. "Besides, don't you think I look quite captivating as Lady Marian?"

"Spare me!" Leander said.

"And if the truth be told, Leander, you make a most handsome Robin Hood. But that's not all. I have a secret to tell you."

"What is it?" Leander said.

"Oh no—I don't sell my secrets so cheaply."

"That's not fair!"

"My price is a promise you'll return to the party."

"NO!"

"Fine, no promise, no secret. I'm leaving. You bore me."

"All right you win. You know I can't resist a secret. What is it?"

"Your Father has bought you the most wonderful madras silk cravat. The very one you most admired when last we were on the Strand."

"I've made quite a mess of it, haven't I?" Leander said, begging for reassurance against reproach.

"Don't be a goose," said Pandora. "You've done no such thing. You played your part almost flawlessly and if we get back right away, there won't be any to-do about it."

"You're saying that only as a vain attempt to placate me. You know I was completely absurd." Leander drew himself in and went back to his book. Pandora just sat there, silently waiting, dangling her feet through the railing, watching the young man hunched over, trying to shut her out.

"What do you mean, 'almost flawlessly'?" Leander said, finally.

"Well," Pandora returned, moving quickly toward the discarded cap, "I would have preferred your hat a little more to one side." And with that she placed it at a rakish angle on his head. "There, now you are perfect!"

She leaned close to him and let her hands rest on his shoulders. Leander put his arms around her waist and gently drew her to him.

"Lady Marian...?" he said.

"Yes, Robin."

"I think I love you."

She felt the brim of his hat go through her hair as their lips met in the sweetness of a first kiss.

CHAPTER SEVENTEEN

General Miranda was a victim of an irascible affliction. He was a chronic insomniac. On the all too frequent occasions when he could not sleep, it was his custom to dress fully and go to his library, where he would read and write until the torturous night ended, either by the reprieve of dawn or the blessing of slumber.

Tonight he had actually fallen asleep quite easily, only to be awakened by the yowl of a cat in heat. Once roused, there was to be no return. When he reached the gallery leading to the library, his boots registered their imprint against the silence, and Pandora sat up in her bed. Still cuddling her china doll, which had remained the final vestige of her childhood, she paused for a moment to gain her bearings.

The room was brimful of the acquirements of the past years. Books lined the walls, making allowance on occasion for a well placed keepsake given to her by Leander. Clothes were everywhere, having outgrown their drawers and armoire, their bright colors signifying, like a clarion horn, Pandora's coming of age—a young girl, not quite a woman, but clearly no longer a child. She reached for her dressing gown and knitted shawl, then made her way in the dark, down the stairs to await the general.

This had become a ritual, the general trying to be as quiet as possible so as not to waken her, while she set the snare by leaving her door ajar to be sure and hear his approach. Therefore it was no wonder that, however painstaking his stealth, most nights Miranda would find the sleepy girl waiting for him at the bottom of the stairs.

After carefully closing the door, the general went as usual to light the little fire Topham had laid for him and, as he had come to expect, there was Pandora, yawning and rubbing sleep from her eyes. "How is it that you are still awake?" he asked casually as he lit the fire.

"Oh, I just couldn't sleep," she lied.

"You know, my dear, sleep is an essential tonic for a young lady's beauty." It irritated her that he always responded to the opening parry in this way, drawing a phrase from the common wisdom, and she knew that soon he was bound to apprize her as to the lateness of the hour and the deleterious effects a lack of sleep has on a maiden's constitution. However, just underneath this veneer, she always knew that he was cheered by her presence.

"Did you lay very still and count by threes backwards?" he asked.

"By threes and odds and evens as well," she replied. "It was of no use whatsoever."

"Well, nonetheless," the general said. "March right back upstairs and give it another go. I'm sure you'll succeed!"

By his tone Pandora suspected tonight was not one of those when the general would hold fast to his word. But there were times, during devilish sieges, when one sleepless night had turned to many and the usually gregarious general would be morbid and seek succor in solitude. On those nights he would stand firmly by his edicts and send her back to her room. So when she saw the general settle into his Savonorola chair and take up a book, she knew her assumptions regarding his mood this night were correct and with considerable relief she spoke.

"General Miranda, I have a proposal to make. Suppose I sit over here by the fire and read my book. Then when my eyelids begin to droop, I promise I will go to bed straight away without the least little fuss."

"All right," the general said, not leaving his pages. "But if you are not asleep within the hour, you will go upstairs whether your eyelids are drooping or not."

"Fair enough." She enjoyed this customary bartering, but once a bargain was struck she upheld her end to the letter. This quiet time alone with the general was very special to her and she would do nothing to jeopardize it. "You know, General," she began after a while, "today I was thinking about Mademoiselle Peliciàn, and I was wondering how she is. It has been quite some time since we have received any word from her. I do hope she is fine."

"Well, you certainly have a woman's intuition," the general said, taking a letter from his folio. "You couldn't have asked this question at a more propitious time, for this very evening I received a courier from France, who as per my instructions, had stopped by Rue Menilmontant to see the dear Peliciàn and to make sure she wants for nothing. He informed me that she was in her usual fine fettle, and of course had asked after you. She wondered how you've grown and most particularly if your mind and tongue had slowed down a bit with the passing of time."

Pandora sat listening, all tucked in under her night dress.

"I sent back word assuring her you are becoming a fine young woman, regardless of the fact that your hyperbolic rhythm more resembles a hummingbird than the placid calm of a proper English maiden, and that your passions render you far too romantic for this Anglican Isle. But I dare say," he continued, turning back to his writing, "the poor woman must be in quite a state of agitation now that First Consul Bonaparte has declared himself her Emperor. Do you know my dear, I just realized it is almost ten years to the day, since our first meeting."

Pandora did not react to this observation. She saw no purpose in discussing her past.

"May I ask to whom you are writing?" she said.

"To an American named Madison. We were comrades in arms during their war for independence and he now occupies the office of Secretary of State. Since I expect to be going to America soon, I am arranging to see him on my visit."

"Am I to go?" she asked. *Leaving? America?* She was torn. This was not at all like the last time. Now there was Leander, Mr. Barry, the magnificent library, her beautiful room and wonderful clothes, the theater, the parties, Sarah, Topham, and the others. She realized this had become home and though she still felt her obligation was to be by the general's side, she did not want to leave England.

"No. I'm afraid not. This is a journey involving secret matters and a fair degree of danger, too severe for anyone so tender."

"General, may I remind you," she said with annoyance, "that

though my years be tender, I have already stood well my slice of danger?"

"Your courage will be called upon soon enough, Pandora. And when I have succeeded in my endeavor to free Venezuela, which I assure you as there is a God in Heaven that I will, then you will join me and together we will build the 'New Republic of Colombia,' a nation the likes of which this blessed earth has never seen. Till that day you must continue your studies and prepare for the great adventure which lies ahead. For in our new society, each one can be whatever their abilities will allow."

"But what am I to prepare for? How will I serve you in Colombia?"

"In Colombia," the general began, "you can be whatever your imagination envisions. The only barriers you will encounter are those produced by the limits of your capabilities. And I dare say my child, in your case, only God knows where those barriers lie."

Pandora grew very silent and covered her face up with her book. The general came over and stood behind her high-backed chair, resting his hands on its wings.

"I have this awful feeling deep inside," she said, "that you're never coming back. That we'll never be together in Colombia, and that you'll die there all alone, without me."

"Now I want you to listen to me very carefully," he said, as they both stared straight ahead into the fire. "All things must die, for that is the order of nature. Death must not attract your concern, it manages its own affairs. The force of life, that is what you must focus upon. Your raison d'etre. That must be the object of your mind, your passion and your will. Only God decides how many days you will have. But how you fill those days is up to you. So if I am to die in the service of a noble mission—shed no tears for me." He kissed her lightly on the forehead and patted her hand.

"I'm sorry for becoming so sullen," she said.

"Don't be foolish, such swings of mood are an irresistible part of a young lady's charm. Now I must finish my correspondence."

Pandora looked down at the pages of her open book, the general's words turning over and over in her head. The fire warmed her against the nights chill, and the constant scratching of Miranda's quill calmed her. Soon the words on the page blurred, her lids became heavy and her head dropped.

She was transformed into a bird flying high above the earth, one of a great flock, bound in tight formation on their migratory journey. Looking down, she saw beneath the coastline of Venezuela, just as it had appeared on the general's maps. Over the shoals they came, searching the clear water for fish. As they neared the beach, soaring upward on the warm winds, Pandora smelled smoke and heard the sounds of a gunshot. The flock veered in one motion away from the shore and its foreboding noises, but she started down, separating herself from the rest.

When she landed on the blood soaked sand, she saw that she was surrounded by heads scattered willy-nilly about the beach. But no matter where she looked, the burning eyes of those severed heads fixed themselves on her. As a bird everything was of larger scale for her and she had to keep fluttering up and down between the debris of heads and discarded props of battle.

All at once she came upon the bodies that belonged to these many heads. They were all lined up in a row in a sitting position, their muskets raised and pointing toward the brush which bordered the beach. Pandora hopped up onto the butt of one of the raised muskets to enhance her view, when suddenly from the bushes came a scream so violent and wrathful she almost lost her bearing and had to beat her wings to regain position.

In a flurry of crashing metal and giant sweeping motions, General Miranda charged onto the beach and tore across the sand toward the enemy's position. His face was twisted into such a contortion that Pandora might not have recognized him were it not for her familiarity with him. The cry that had drawn her attention away from the enemy fire was of such rage it seemed the general would tear his throat.

Pandora opened her beak to call a warning to the general but nothing emerged. She pushed hard from her neck but nothing happened. She flapped her wings, trying to rise from her perch, but her clawed feet were clamped in an iron grip around the muzzle of the gun. "Don't go! Don't go! You mustn't go! You mustn't go! Please, please don't go!" she finally screamed, her own voice coming to her. Her feet began to pull away from the gun but she could not fly and fell to the ground with a hard thud. When she opened her eyes she saw she was on the floor next to her bed with half of her covers around her. She looked up at the window and saw the first light of dawn breaking the night sky. The general must have carried her up. She looked around her in the dim light of dawn and realized she was alone.

CHAPTER EIGHTEEN

There was no further possibility of sleep. Her mind was abuzz, the general's challenge repeating itself over and over. Finally, she made for her secret hiding place underneath the bottom drawer of her dresser, where she had sequestered the black tin box Mademoiselle Pelicièn had given her. She lay it on her lap and opened it slowly, pulling out Mademoiselle's handkerchief, which held the ebony rosary beads with the gold crucifix. Pandora put the hanky up to her nose and filled her head with Mademoiselle's earthy scent. Then she draped the rosary around her wrist, putting the cross between her thumb and forefinger. At once she began to rub the emaciated figure of Jesus with her thumb, then closing her eyes, she prayed, "If You are truly here, if You really do exist as the Son of God, I ask with pure heart and soul that You show yourself to me, and I will follow You in whatever direction You so give." She waited a while for some materialization and when none was forthcoming, she reasoned that a visitation might be too much to expect, since she was so unpracticed at prayer.

Again she raised the hanky to her nose and this time breathed three times. "All right then, I merely request a small sign. Nothing big, perhaps a picture falling from the wall or a little bird pecking at my window, or a small ray of light on my pillow." She sat very still and concentrated with all her power while she ardently rubbed the figure, repeating again and again, "Please, God, please, God, please, God, please, God." But the room was attendant with only the silences of the summer morning. "All right then, if that's the way You want it!"

She bolted up, bounded onto her bed and raised the little cross to heaven. "If I am not worthy of Your blessing, then let me at least feel the sting of Your curses." She squeezed tight the cross until her arm began to tremble, "Damn You! I knew You wouldn't come! I knew You wouldn't help me! Why didn't You help the children under the bridge and the poor people in the prisons? Why didn't You help my mother? She must have begged You. If you didn't help us, then who do You help?!" She cocked back her arm to fling the crucifix, but was stopped by the sight of her own image in the mirror. She ran to her reflection and shook the frame. "I don't need any God! I'll do it all by myself." Then, with a cold expression and a defiant posture, she sat at her desk and began to list, with unsettling objectivity, her three greatest attributes.

"My ability to retain and recall in precise detail any event—no matter if it be read or witnessed." She dipped her pen in the ink, and scratched out the second, "Indefatigable determination." But this next one, she thought, is the most important. Leaving a big space, she wrote in broad hand, "M'etudiant, my studying." She had called it this as far back as she could remember. It referred to her ability to switch all of her mental gears in one direction simultaneously, unhampered by fear and without concern for consequence. This gave her the facility to examine an individual or situation in its entirety and see coldly and precisely all that is involved—a level of inspection that the cleverest of guises or pretensions could not veil. She performed this rite constantly and naturally. It came to her as easily as breath, though she was aware that with consistent use it had improved, becoming sharper and more refined.

Not only had it always been her sole means of self-defense, but also her favorite pastime, an unending source of pleasure and power. She leaned back in her chair and held up the paper to blow the ink dry. Encouraged by her work, she returned to her deliberations, deciding now that she had brought her best qualities to light she should try to match them to an appropriate calling. Starting again with a fresh sheet, she made a list of the five learned professions and prepared to explore each in its turn.

She went to her wardrobe and took the black opera cape from it. She pinned any wayward curls securely to the top of her head, then threw the cape in one grand sweep over her shoulders and exited her room to the balcony rail.

"Gentlemen!" she shouted."Look carefully at this man whose life you would take, whose wife you would widow, whose children you would deny the strong hand of a good and loving father. Then ask yourselves one simple question." She paused only long enough to wheel on her imaginary jury.

"What, pray you, is the proof of evidence against him?" She pointed an accusatory finger at them.

"Pandora!"

She started and turned to the rail again.

"Leander, have you been sitting there all of this time?"

"Long enough to wonder whether you'd been working on a play to perform—or just gone mad."

"Leander, do you think these people," she motioned toward her imaginary jury, "would be able to separate the innocent from the guilty even with a brilliant summation? After all, they might be nothing but fools, barbarians thirsting for punishment, blinded from the truth by prejudice, incapable of properly adjudicating any case despite crystal clarity and simplicity of definition. Oh no, Leander!" She flung her arms over the railing with a broad theatrical gesture.

"I will never break through such barriers of irrationality. The law is not for me!"

She sat hard on the floor and leaned her head on the rail post.

"Pandora," Leander asked, "What in the devil's name are you talking about?"

"Oh!" She popped up and started down the circular stair.

"Last night, I had the most important talk with General Miranda and he told me about his mission to free Venezuela and to build the Republic of Colombia and how we can be all that we want to be there. All that stands in our way is timidity of imagination or lack of capability." She noticed Leander did not show one ounce of enthusiasm concerning what she just said.

"Well," she prodded, "have you been listening or are you in another world—your usual place."

"Indeed not!" Leander snapped. "I would venture to say it is you who has left this solid plane. Sit down," he said, "and listen to me."

Pandora sat on the bottom stair.

"All my life I have listened to my father talk of his 'New Republic of Colombia.' All my life he has disappeared for years at a time, sometimes mysteriously, always suddenly and always with the promise that this time when he returns we would be departing with him to the new republic where we could be all that we need to be."

Leander's imitative gesture and sarcastic tone rankled Pandora.

"Every corner of this house is filled with the illusions of his 'mission.' Pandora, there is no Colombia for him or for us, and the proof is clear. Nothing has ever come of his tall tales."

"How dare you! What an insufferable prig you are. How dare you question him." Pandora bolted up. "Where have you been, what have you done that gives you just cause for such skepticism. You have never left this house, your cocoon, your protection. So you don't see anything. You're just a caterpillar waiting, asleep in your chrysalis; you'll never be a butterfly!"

She did not wait for Leander's response, she ran to her room and flung herself on her bed.

"Don't you run away from me." Leander charged into her room, his full black brow arched in a fierce expression, his eyes glowing.

"You think life is just one long escapade. One moment you are filling your head with wild dreams, adventures, the next you are off to live them out regardless of whether they are based on fantasy or reality. Well, let me tell you, 'Miss Dream World,' that is not at all the stuff of life. What is going on before your eyes is what life is about. Real adventure emerges out of that. Dreams come true out of that. Love comes out of that. But you have no idea what I'm talking about because all you want to do is make up things and then convince yourself that they are true."

"You don't seem to understand, Leander, you're missing the point entirely. It doesn't matter whether the general's dream is real or not. He took me in off the streets of Paris and changed my fate, and for that I have a sacred obligation to serve him in whatever way I can."

"Sacred obligation! That's very noble indeed. Is that why you're dressing up and deluding yourself with notions of law, because of a sacred obligation? Well, now I know you can't be thinking straight! You're a woman, Pandora, and you should see what 'sacred obligations' you're going to have as such."

"I don't need you to tell me who I am and how I should think. I suppose you would prefer if I only thought about you. Well, that would really be frivolous."

Leander's back was already disappearing through the door.

"Leand—!" she stopped herself. What could she say to soften those hateful words. She threw the cape against the wall. So what, he deserved it, he asked for it. Reality, you don't know what it is. She mocked him, but suddenly, without warning, tears sprung to her eyes and a terrible feeling of loss or emptiness weighed her down. She went and lay on her bed and let the tears fall into her ears and run down her jawbone. She had hurt him.

She thought about how they had sat together at night so close together they could count each other's breathing, how she always watched him pretend he was concentrating on his book, but she knew he was just waiting to be sure all the family had retired for the night so that he could take her hand. With feminine cunning she had always played her part and let it rest casually atop her skirts. But every time he took it she would feel a shiver of surprise and excitement run through her and her breath would catch and she'd let out a self-conscious giggle. It never failed to be this way even though she always knew exactly what was going to happen.

Now she had stabbed him with her words and he'd never wait for her to take her place, to hold her hand, or to quickly, sweetly touch her lips with his before he ran off to his room. She'd ruined everything. How could she repair it? He loved her.

CHAPTER NINETEEN

As the months wore on Pandora's predicament remained unsolved. Not only were her waking hours disrupted, but even her sleep had brought her no respite. Each night she was visited by intense dreams, so lucid that for moments after she awoke she would not know whether they were real. Because of their disturbing nature, she knew they must hold some key, so she always wrote them down in a special book with as meticulous a memory as possible. But to date this had proved no help to her and, try as she might, she could not glean any clues from them. Finally, she realized she needed to talk to someone and there was only one person she knew to whom she could confide her dreams, her teacher, James Barry.

Why, he was perfect. She could trust his solemn word without precaution. Above and beyond every other consideration she had come to see that, despite his eccentric and somewhat boisterous style, his wisdom abounded, and he had a poet's way of seeing. Many was the time she heard his words in her ear long after they'd been spoken. With solid resolve she headed up the narrow twisting stairway to his garret under the roof.

When James Barry heard the light knocking at his door, he was mildly surprised. It had become practice, though never a rule, that when the painter withdrew to his rooms, he was not to be disturbed. Thus he knew that any such interruption could only signal a matter of importance.

Approaching the door, his heart beating in rapid anticipation of unsettling news, he shot a quick look at his wet canvas before opening. Pandora stood there, book in hand, a most downcast look on her face.

Barry had been worried by the steady change in her temper of late and was particularly vexed by the animosity and coldness she displayed toward Leander, from whom he could extract no explanation. Nor could he himself succeed in warming their relations. Finally, he had accepted the situation and allowed his two pupils to participate in their studies as if in fact they were doing so in separate rooms. Finding Pandora in his doorway, obviously ready and wanting to talk, put him in the best of humor. Any resentment or anger he might have felt upon the first sounds of intrusion were forgiven.

"I know that this is the time you are usually occupied with your painting, sir. I hope you will excuse the interruption and forgive my ill manners," Pandora said.

"Think nothing of it, my dear. Your timing is actually impeccable. I've had no luck at all this afternoon prodding recalcitrant muses and was just about to pack it up. So why don't you come in and sit down, for you appear to be in an eager state."

Pandora entered and settled herself on the edge of the long chaise upon which Barry often catnapped between energetic sessions with his canvasses. "Would you care for an apple?" he asked.

"No thank you, sir."

"Well that's fine. No food, just conversation. Everyone knows how much I love a good talk. Now, what is it that has brought you here?"

Pandora sat ordering her thoughts for a moment and the artist took advantage of the time to study her face and see how it was maturing.

"I have a request before we begin," she said. "I would beg that this conversation be kept between the two of us."

"You need not trouble yourself about that for one instant, my dear lady. You are speaking to the very soul of discretion. Why, between these two rather protrusive ears are held some of the great secrets of all Britain, which, no amount of torture will ever force past my lips."

In spite of herself, Pandora laughed at her teacher's stylish proclamation, and the tension which she had carried in with her lightened.

Turning the easel toward the wall, Barry winked. "Just so. I will not be distracted by its beckoning," he said.

"As you know, Mr. Barry," Pandora began, "the general is soon to launch his expedition to Venezuela. I must be prepared to the fullest of my capabilities to take my place in this new republic, in order to both realize its dream and express the depth of my gratitude to the general, and I must structure this commitment into a concrete form, a choice of profession."

Suddenly part of the picture became clear to him. In the past months Pandora had reached such a state of intensity with regard to her studies that even he had thought her obsessive. She would deliver all that he assigned from the day's lessons and return the next ravenous for more, compelling him to feed, with rapid dispatch, her never ending hunger for new material. He had not seen that the "sacred mission" of General Miranda was the driving force behind her behavior. But even this did not explain her bitter and venomous attitude toward Leander, which had soured the teacher's full pleasure of her achievements.

"I'll get right to the point," Pandora continued, in the same determined way. "The general has told me I can be anything possible in the new world, as long as I am prepared. But no matter how hard I try to see what it is I am best suited for, and in which vocation I would be the most helpful, I keep walking down blind alleys which lead nowhere. I am at an impasse. I have made lists of all my strengths and weaknesses, and have tried to match them to various professions, but to no avail. And now I have become desperate. You see, Mr. Barry, I cannot idle away my time with unfocused pursuit any longer. I know that the general could be leaving at any time. He is only awaiting word from friends in America and now that we are soon to be at war with Spain, why it is certain the English will become our allies. So you see I have no time to lose."

Pandora's earnestness and sincerity touched Barry deeply, but he was disturbed to realize that her attachment to General Miranda was not that of an orphan to a substitute father but rather that of a supplicant toward a savior.

"Pandora," Barry said, "why do you come to me? How can I possibly help you? Politics and revolution, as you well know, are not my specialty. I am only able to teach you from the classical wisdom of the past, which has endured to the present. I know very little of this bold new world you and the general envision..." He stopped short for he was about to call attention to the general's human imperfections. He knew better, but Pandora did not seem to notice his abrupt hesitation.

"Remember the other day? When we were reading from the dialogues of Plato, Socrates was speaking to Phaedrus of the difference between sanity and madness?" Pandora said.

"Ah, yes," Barry said, beginning to grasp what the intention of the visit might be. "I surmise you have come to me seeking clarity on the third type of madness, of which Socrates spoke. A possession of the muses!" Barry began to recite from memory, "But he who, not being inspired and having no touch of madness in his soul, if he thinks he will get into the temple by the help of art, he, I say, and his poetry, will not be admitted. So!" Barry exclaimed, standing now with a self-satisfied expression on his face. "You have come to your old teacher, knowing that he is a little bit mad and thinking his madness may succeed where sanity has failed. I am stating it correctly, am I not, dear girl?"

"No sir, not at all. I do not think you the least bit mad but rather an artist who has a level of perception others lack. I have brought with me this book in which I have recorded my dreams as accurately as I was able. I had hoped you could glean some hint of inspiration which might shed light on my predicament."

Barry took the notebook from the child's hand and sat down to read, only stopping on occasion for some clarification since Pandora's handwriting, like her hair, tended toward the wild. He read until the candle had burned to the nub. Pandora never moved. She sat in sober silence awaiting his response. Finally, he put the book aside, rose and stretched his back. "Well, I don't know if this will be of any use to you," he said rubbing his neck, "but they all tell the same tale, don't they?"

Pandora looked quizzically at him. "I don't know what you mean."

"A mere change of buttons on the frock, but each is always of the same weave. In each dream you are constantly surrounded by people who are hurt, in pain or are, for some reason in dire need of your aid. You have no idea how to comfort them, yet you yearn to do so. In each dream you are being called upon to change their condition, or in some way give back what they have lost...."

"You mean, as in the dream with the birds?" Pandora said.

"Yes, precisely, here are all the birds—having lost their ability to fly—and they come to you to return it to them. To make it right again. Poetically, one might say, they ask to be returned to their former state of grace."

"I see," she said, an exuberance beginning to charge into her deflated figure. "Like putting the heads back on the soldiers' bodies in the other dream. To put them back together again, to return them to the best, to the proper state. I see now!" She nearly sang her delight which grew with each enlightened thought. "But it's not their souls they want me to fix. No, it's not putting their souls in a proper state, nor is it their minds. No, no, no, it's their bodies. I see it! I see it! How could I have been so blind to miss it? I am to fix their bodies, to cure them. It's so absurdly simple and I missed it."

"What on earth are you talking about?" Barry broke in. "You've lost me entirely. Please slow yourself down a bit so I can understand all of this enthusiasm."

"Oh! Surely you must see it Mr. Barry. It is as clear as day. I just needed you to break the code for me. I am to be a doctor!" she said, laughing out loud at this wonderful notion, "and give people back what they have lost!"

"Well, now!" Barry opened the window and let in the fresh outdoors. "I am happy if I have lessened your burden, but now I would like you to answer me a question. What on earth has transpired between you and Leander? And what does it have to do with your obligation to General Miranda?"

Immediately, Pandora lost her sense of elation and looked away from Mr. Barry. "I'm sorry, sir," she said. "That situation is one of such privacy I cannot discuss it with anyone." She rose to leave.

"Very well, Pandora, I will probe no further. But may I leave you with one thought? The thematic material of your dreams has to do with making others whole. Perhaps it is you who needs to be made whole and that may have far more to do with Leander than with the general."

CHAPTER TWENTY

"It's the most preposterous idea I have ever heard, completely and utterly ludicrous. Why, I would no more stand before the board of trustees of Edinburgh University and advocate the admission of a woman into its medical school than I would jump off the London Bridge!"

The Earl of Buchan rose from his chair, his face growing red as he spoke, until finally he had to dab at his forehead more than once, as heavy moisture began to form there and increase with his tirade. "My dear general, as you know I deeply admire your spirit of equality and delight at your shocking even the most complacent listener, this idea rests on the border of madness." Sitting hard in the chair, he adjusted the ruffs on his vest and fanned himself vigorously with his damp handkerchief. The warmth of Lord Buchan's reaction to his proposal immediately made clear to the general that he had greatly miscalculated the character of his ally.

He rose from his chair and stood at attention, a posture he often took in order to control his own volcanic temper.

"My dear sir," he said. "Your heated opposition quite astounds me. For is it not you who so champions the equality of women with your lengthy articles which always emphasize the essentials of education? And are you not the man who said one can judge the level of a civilization by the way its women are treated? Indeed my lord, if I am correct in my recollection, then your reaction to my proposal is in stark contradiction to all that you say you stand for. I must admit this equivocation leaves me in a state of profound confusion."

Above them, her eye pressed to her bedroom door and the tiny crack she'd set, Pandora spied on the souring scene below. Ever since that late night when she'd come down to the library and sprung the news of her decision on the general, he had been captivated.

"The first woman doctor, wouldn't that be something?" he'd said, his eyes mirroring the glow of pride she'd felt upon making the announcement. "Of course, you are aware there is a major obstacle. After all, no where in the world is there or has there ever been a female pupil in a medical school. Nonetheless, my girl, this is truly a bold and audacious idea, and I think it is just grand."

After a quick circumnavigation of the library he had returned to his chair with a smile of satisfaction. "I have a friend and supporter who is first cousin to King George," he said. "He is also on the board of Edinburgh Medical School and is somewhat obsessed with the entire issue of feminine education. Yes, indeed," Miranda had nearly crowed with delighted self-assurance. "The Earl of Buchan holds the key, and if I can persuade him—"

***

"Now, now Francisco," Pandora heard Buchan say, as he shifted uneasily in his chair. He looked for support from James Barry and Leander, who sat opposite him at the other side of the long table. "Of course I am the very same man whom you so accurately described. But as has been true in the past, our point of departure here is not one of ideology but methodology."

Calmed by his own rebuttal, Lord Buchan regained some of his lost composure. He was a man in his prime, unusually tall, standing well over six feet, his legs making the better part of his size. He had a bushy Scottish brow and a coarse thick head of curly brown hair. His clothes were well tailored, skillfully hiding his awkwardness, the result of his length.

"My friend, we are both advocates of the advancement and education of women. But, as is the case in all of these far-reaching and unpopular ideas, I have felt a gradual approach serves a better end. I have never been able to persuade you, my good fellow, that time is primary and will not be defeated by anyone's revolution. We must pursue our goals by extending the limits of our present structures and community standards. That is why I expound my beliefs under a nom de plume. I have learned that when my ideas are presented unaccompanied by my station, it is then and only then that they can be truly heard. In order to make genuine change in a society one needs artfulness more than bravura. A mature man must realize we live in the world that currently exists, not the one of our dreams. Therefore it is my opinion this is not yet the year to propose a woman as a candidate to our most prestigious medical school. Nor do I feel it is the time for such a proposal to be made anywhere. Indeed I am somewhat dismayed that you could be so presumptuous as to try to impose such a weight on me. I have been eager to support you in other areas and no one is happier than I to see that your expedition to South America is finally at hand. But this request pushes me beyond my limit."

Miranda tried to interject but Lord Buchan, waving his hand, would not be dissuaded.

"No, General Miranda, one cannot supersede the conventions of time no matter one's will. In one hundred years hence, I am sure the universities of the world will be filled with women. But you and I will long be dead and gone."

Pandora's heart sank. She knew the general had lost any firm ground from which to turn Lord Buchan around. And Leander's contained but victorious smile was more than she could bear.

"Gentlemen!" she called. "May I be so bold as to interject a word or two on my own behalf?" She moved quickly down the stairs in order to stave off a negative response. Her lovely printed afternoon dress accentuating her youthful movement, and the odd strands of her stylishly arranged hair bounced pertly about her resolute face.

"I beg your forgiveness, General Miranda, but I quite agree with Lord Buchan," she said, taking a calculated position of authority at the head of the table next to General Miranda. Lord Buchan gave the general a smile of resolution and leaned triumphantly against the back of his chair. But in a savvy glance Miranda conveyed to Pandora that despite a dismal outlook, he'd not given up, and her intrusion was welcome.

"Clearly, now is not the time for a woman to be admitted to university, but if you will forgive my boldness and immodesty, I must state in front of my honored teacher James Barry, that my education cannot be matched by the most thoroughly prepared medical student in all Britain. My Greek and Latin are flawless, my classics securely in order, and due to the kind acquisition by General Miranda of a fine medical library, I am versed in depth from Celssus to Jenner."

"My dear young woman, I trust absolutely all that you say as truth. Why, your progress has inspired us all and elicited my personal respect and admiration. You are the living proof that a woman's brain is at least equal to that of a man. But I am deeply sorry that there is nothing I can do other than extend my esteem along with my regrets. I am afraid, young lady, you were born a little too soon."

"Lord Buchan," Pandora said, "have you heard of a scientific principle, referred to as Occam's Razor?"

"No," he responded, "I don't believe I have ever heard of such an axiom, but I fail to see—?"

"Please, sir, if you will give me a moment I will show you clearly what I have in mind. And from there I think it can be accepted that all our previous problems will be solved. Plainly put, Occam's Razor states that given a choice of rival theories, one should always pick the simplest. One which is in accord with all of the facts. In this case we have two conflicting facts. Fact number one, the world has not yet progressed to the point where women anywhere are admitted to university for training. Fact number two, I am most qualified to be a candidate for admission to Edinburgh Medical School. But fact number one cancels out fact number two, because I am a woman. Isn't that correct?"

Everyone nodded.

"But there is a third fact, not to be overlooked. That is, if I were a man—equipped precisely as I am as a woman—would there be any question with regards to your sponsorship of me as a student at Edinburgh for the coming semester?"

"Why, not at all," Lord Buchan declared.

"Fine," Pandora said. "Then it is a clear path. The perfect resolution to our quandary is that I be admitted as a man!"

"Now you're talking like a woman," Buchan chuckled. "You've lost me completely. What on earth do you mean, a man?"

"Come, Lord Buchan." Pandora took General Miranda's ornamental dagger from its cradle and gingerly tested the razor sharp edge with her thumb. "Surely you can see—why it's as plain as your nom de plume." With quick and clean gestures she released one of the fasts holding her hair and before anyone really understood what she was doing she sliced off a handful. "Lord Buchan," she said, dropping the severed curls onto the table. "You put forth your ideas behind another name. I will put mine forth behind another appearance."

The Earl of Buchan threw his head back with a roar of laughter, but when Pandora looked at Leander his face was ripe with disgust.

CHAPTER TWENTY-ONE

"Father, do you think the Emperor Napoleon is really planning to invade England?"

"Well, Leander, it's finally coming to a climax." Miranda peered over the top of his newspaper at his son's long figure stretched on the blue spread neatly laid on the grass of Green Park.

"Then you think there'll be war at any time?" Leander sat upright and squinted in the bright warm sunlight. Pandora watched from her corner near the picnic basket.

"Of this, my son, one should have no doubt. Even without the intelligence reports to which I am privy one needs only understand that a man of his character can never be content with a string full of small fish. Therefore he must attack England and, mark my words, some day in the not so distant future he will march his Grande Armée into Russia.

"But, Father, if we're about to declare war won't that delay your departure?"

"On the contrary, war in Europe will be extremely advantageous to my situation. With Spain fighting alongside the French, their naval resources will be focused on the European arena, leaving Venezuela vulnerable. God willing, I plan to exploit this configuration to its fullest."

Pandora continued listening to them with only half an ear. These days she had been thinking only of herself, her journey to Edinburgh and her admission to its medical school. She had been spending long hours at her Latin and anatomy studies and whatever time she had left she had rigorously gone over the subtleties of her grand masquerade—the walk, the movement of the hands, tilt of the head. In fact, though it was Sunday and beautiful and warm, she had resisted coming along on the picnic when Miranda suggested it. Somehow everything around her had disappeared from her concern other than her own imminent adventure. She barely noticed or cared about Leander's growing coldness and distance from her. The general's machinations barely crossed her mind. The fact that her beloved teacher had begun to hack quite disturbingly from a nagging cough and that his face looked gray had only occupied fleeting moments of awareness. Even the inducement of today's May Day fireworks and the unheard of sight of a man parachuting from a balloon had not whetted her enthusiasm much. But for the sake of familial harmony she had relented.

"Father, you don't think it's possible that that little Corsican weasel could defeat us at sea and succeed with a landed invasion? God, I'd rather be dead than French."

Pandora accepted this barb with an expressionless face. Leander had never shown any love toward her homeland but ever since she had made her decision to go to medical school, his anti-French sentiments knew no bounds. Whenever the slightest opportunity occurred he expressed with shark-toothed sarcasm his distaste for things French. He aimed his sights with precision and care toward areas in which he knew she had particular interest—fashion, food, and politics—then fired hard to hurt her. It had become their only means of communication even though Pandora pretended to be unruffled each time, such as now.

"War, my son, is never predictable," Miranda said, rising from his chair. "And though the French fleet is quite impressive, I have little doubt that the shining strength of the English character, from their admirals right down to their common seamen, will prevail."

As they walked off toward a small pond, Pandora reflected how father and son had drawn closer. It was increasingly clear to her this closeness was between men and she had no place in it.

"Pandora!" Sarah called her. "It's time to stop daydreaming and start eating. Now open the basket, fix yourself a plate and come out of the clouds."

The wind disturbed the wide brim of Sarah's yellow bonnet, creating shadows of light and dark on her face. Pandora was struck by her beauty anew as the altered shades highlighted her features even more. Sarah loved picnics.

Carmen and Rosa returned from their stroll and plunged into the viands and breads they had so carefully prepared. Topham sat snoozing on a wooden recliner, his hat low over his eyes. He sucked in a snore and Pandora smiled at his guileless sleep. She saw no sign of Leander and the general and while they were gone no one spoke of Miranda's voyage West or its close arrival. Nor did they speak of the fact that James Barry was absent. He had agreed after much nagging on Sarah's part to stay in and rest, his condition—the cough and a new wheeze in his chest—having warranted a threat by her of a visit from a doctor. Everyone knew of course he was probably painting furiously behind his closed doors at this very moment.

Suddenly there was a sound of exclamations and huzzahs and a wave of people stood pointing toward the heavens. At the far end of the park a huge balloon appeared. Everyone on the green began to cheer as the great orb covered with a fine net silently drifted toward them, leaving a shadow behind it as it passed over.

"He's going to break his fool neck," Topham said, unhappy to be aroused from his afternoon slumber by all the commotion. "Ain't no one can survive from that height, whatever they so-called parachute down in. It ain't natural. The general may as well have taken us to a good hanging seeing as how that makes more sense than what this fool is about to do."

Pandora picked up the general's binocle and focused in on the coming balloon. She could see a thin dark man working with great haste at his final preparations. He stood inside a substantial, heavy looking basket, from the center of which rose a pole with a large open umbrella attached with many strings to his gondola. The upper part was somehow connected to the bottom of the balloon. It seemed to her it couldn't possibly work—the whole apparatus being much too inelegant and heavy to come down to earth from that great height with anything other than a disastrous result.

"Now, Mr. Topham," General Miranda said, suddenly appearing a bit breathless from out of the crowd with Leander at his side. "Have a little faith in progress and human ingenuity."

Just then the car and giant umbrella were detached from the balloon and in a series of wide swings it began to come toward earth. Everyone ran toward the phenomenal sight as the big balloon, loose strings trailing like a thousand tails behind it, drifted away. A boisterous cheer and a deluge of hats flew into the air as the man in the parachute hit the ground and proudly, though on slightly wobbly legs, waved.

"Imagine this, Leander," Miranda said, competing with the din. "An army of flying balloons dropping soldiers from above, wherever they need them to be and ready to fight.

The jumper, no worse for wear other than a twisted ankle, regained his earth legs and smiled to the captivated audience surrounding him. Immediately several men hoisted him off the ground and carried him aloft to the ringing cheers of the throng. They put him down before the bandstand, and after hopping up the steps with a great show of effort, he turned arms raised in victory as the brass band struck a heraldry in his honor. As the sun was already behind the trees which bordered the far end of the park, everyone returned to their own parties. Soon the glow of lanterns began to fill the park and the cluster of picnickers acquired the romantic glow a painter might capture on his easel. Brightly illuminated in the center of this scene was the gazebo in which the band enthusiastically slid from one tune to another.

"Attention!" Miranda tapped his wine glass. "Now that we've witnessed a modern miracle of courage and technology, enjoyed a fine repast supplied by the ladies of the house, I think it the right time for a proud announcement of my own. My son Leander has secured a commission in the Royal Marines and on the morrow he leaves for Portsmouth. Sarah," he turned to Sarah, whose expression reflected both pride and concern. "We've managed to raise a fine lad, who is bound to bring glory to himself and honor to his family."

A great swooshing sound diverted everyone's attention as a golden cascade of light burst in the sky and fell to oblivion in the quiet distance. The fireworks started just at the right moment. Pandora knew that Leander's recent closeness to his father had to result in some secret and even though she was as proud as Sarah must be, she was hurt that she was kept in the dark about it until now. Upon the general's announcement, her face had begun to burn and a few tears involuntarily escaped. Not daring to look at Leander, she glued herself to the pyrotechnics. Leander was becoming a man and his own man at that. She wanted to put her arms around his neck and cry on his shoulder like any woman whose love was soon to go off to war, but her pride held her fast and she sat feeling isolated and alone under the glorious shower of lights that filled the night sky.

CHAPTER TWENTY-TWO

"Open the curtains!" Barry said, prompting an intense attack of coughing. "Light, I need some light, damn it! Only the most pusillanimous poltroon would take away light from the painter."

"But, Dr. Webster—" Sarah said.

"Damn Dr. Webster! He's a quack, like all the rest. It's a miracle if anyone gets well under their care. The art of science and medicine, that's an oxymoron if ever there was one." Barry glared at Pandora who was sitting by him, an open book on her lap. She ignored his not so subtle barb. With resignation Sarah threw open the opaque drapes and a flood of sunshine spread over the room, warming everything except the hideously ashen color of James Barry's face.

"Let me help you sit up." Pandora pulled him forward and stuffed as many pillows behind him as she could. He was very thin and tremulously weak.

In the beginning, lots of tea and at least one strongly-resisted mustard plaster had been given with some relief. But against all advice he had continued to paint all day and go off into the damp nights to his favorite haunts to argue with his usual fervor about the nature of art with anyone who'd listen. A week ago, he had come home soaked to the bone from a heavy rain. His eyes were glazed from fever. "I couldn't pay for a carriage. I spent all my money on some new canvases," he had shouted at Sarah, who, though frightened by his near delirium, scolded him for walking home in a downpour.

A doctor had been summoned immediately and pronounced

that Barry was now suffering from an acute abscess of the lung, complicated by his weakened condition. A result of his stubborn resistance to earlier advice and treatment, the doctor could not promise an optimistic outcome. As the week wore on, it was clear to all James Barry was dying.

General Miranda was in the final stages of preparation for his South American expedition and had been spending almost all his time sequestered in the library going over papers, correspondence, and the securing of his crew and supplies. But every day he interrupted his large efforts and came to visit his ailing friend, always entering with an effervescent energy and a jovial word.

"General Miranda," Pandora said, softly interrupting his hunched-over concentration.

"Has there been any change in his condition?" Miranda sat up and put down the quill.

"While his spirit still soars, the body is failing fast," she said, her lack of sleep showing.

"I spoke with Dr. Webster yesterday afternoon," Miranda said. "He anticipates it won't be long. I've sent for Leander. What time is it?"

"Just after three," she said.

"Well, he should be here any moment." Miranda opened the library door. "Now let's go to the old fellow."

Pandora stepped first into the hallway.

"It seems like we're all leaving you one way or another, Pandora," Miranda said, putting his arm around her shoulder.

"Yes sir, it does seem so."

"You know, I fully expect before long you and I will be back together to begin the greatest of our adventures, but if God has something else in mind..." By now they had reached Mr. Barry's door. "I would like to leave you with a thought. No matter what the cost or consequence, one must be true to and fight for the highest ideals. That means that one must put personal desires behind the needs of history and that, above all else, service must take precedence over self. It is a high mountain to climb but it is the way to the top." He kissed her forehead. "From the first day I met you I knew you were special. Your path will be lonesome and sometimes sad but I have no doubt you will do great good."

Barry still sat propped straight up in his bed, his breathing labored. Leander stood at the foot. He wore a short scarlet jacket, white crossed belt over his chest. His britches were sharp white and in the crook of his arm he held his high, rounded hat. Miranda went over and shook his hand firmly.

"I have something to say," Barry said, looking at Leander, the general and Pandora.

"Perhaps you should just rest, sir," Leander said.

"Don't patronize me. I can see through you and that silly uniform like glass. Rest will be my total occupation in a very short time, so let me say my piece before I'm no longer able." He began to cough violently. Simultaneously, Pandora and Leander rushed to either side of his bed and lifted him higher to try and quell the attack. Their eyes met. Leander's were warm and full. Pandora attempted to wipe Barry's mouth with a handkerchief but he waved her off irritably.

"Sit down, sit down, let me be." He patted the bed on either side. "Good," he said, taking each of their hands. "It's been a long time since I've seen you two this close together. As you well know I am not a church man, but I do believe in God and that there exists a divine pattern in all things. I have spent my life as a painter trying to see that pattern and to share it with others. Since I can no longer put a brush to canvas I am going to tell you what I see."

"Leander, I know that you love Pandora and that she loves you as well, though of late neither of you has admitted this to himself or the other. I see that there will be many times to come where this love will meet strange and unexpected twists and turns and perhaps seem broken. But whatever forces brought you together, the bond has been sewn too strongly to break. You must always remember it is a holy connection. It is inescapable. It is destiny." Barry joined their hands together, then he looked straight ahead at General Miranda.

CHAPTER TWENTY-THREE

The October rain fell in a gentle mist, darkening the straw covers which hung from the scaffolds affronting the old buildings of Edinburgh University, and the air was filled with their musky smell. Pandora marched under the huge archway towards the bursar's office, her footsteps gaining momentum as she passed through the ranks of laborers industriously engaged, despite the mornings rain. Hod carriers climbed stalwart ladders, sure-handed carpenters plied their trade and powerfully built men wielded heavy sledges. This great university had endured more than two hundred years, but of late her labors had been slowed and hampered by the exigencies of time. Buildings of the seventeenth century no longer suited the needs of the infant nineteenth. So despite the resistance of tradition and the reluctant spending of a penny-pinching town board, change came. Unwelcome by some, inconvenient to all, it filled the air with its dust.

Pandora pulled the collar of her overcoat high around her chin and ran her gloved hand against the nape of her neck, touching the ends of her cropped curls. This was her first venture into public as a man, her premier appearance. At the outset she had experienced a certain light-headedness, which increased somewhat when she encountered the workmen. But she attributed this to the effects of the tight bindings around her breasts, which undoubtedly inhibited her breathing. Setting her course across the quad, she headed in a direct line toward the bursar's door. But with each successive step her anxiety intensified. At first it only affected her legs, forcing her to concentrate hard on her objective. Then her entire body began to feel as if it were no longer subject to her command and she thought for sure, at any moment, she would faint.

She had, she thought, prepared herself well for the masquerade. In the beginning she had studied the men around her, watching them with unbroken concentration. The way they spoke and laughed, how they stood and sat, the way they crossed and uncrossed their legs and, most important, how they were with each other and how they were with women. Each day she chose one element of behavior to work on; removing herself to the solitude of the library, she had attempted to alter this element within herself. A day's work may have been spent on her walk, pitch and manner of speech, or on a particularly masculine activity such as cigar smoking or billiards. Whichever it was, she carried on these exercises with supreme diligence. Therefore it wasn't too long a time before she realized these machinations were both absurd and futile. No matter what the effort, her appearance remained unalterably that of a petite young girl only trying some grotesque attitudes of maleness.

Then one day, while observing Topham's coarse manner and attempting a like gruffness to her voice, she came to a rather startling and profound discovery. Not all men were the same. In Topham's case, everything was on a massive scale, suitable to his size. But in the case of Leander, for example, it was quite a different story. That difference held the key to her new character. Leander, though tall, was thin like herself, he was temperamental, as was she and always ready to use a sharp tongue and quick wit in response to any affront. At that moment she saw the obvious. She would never convince anyone she was a typical rough and tumble lad, a man's man. No, she would have to convince the world she was a youth of a highly strung countenance, tinged with eccentricities, captured in a small body. This then would become the guiding principle, in which she would put her faith for success. She would change herself as little as possible, only cropping her hair and adopting a name and costume, which the superficial observer would see as the accouterments of a sensitive young man.

Now for the first time her hypotheses were really being tested. The perspiration which had welled up under her bindings, began to run down her rib cage, making damp spots on the chemise under her coat. What in the name of God am I doing, she thought, doubt nurturing her anxiety. Just then she was startled by a solid pounding on the back. "New here?" a voice queried. She turned to confront a very tall and rather foppish young man smiling broadly down at her. He was nattily dressed. Pandora noticed right off his splendid ascot, pinned high on the throat.

"Palmer, Robin Penwell," the young man continued with another strong double tap on the back. She could tell by his haughty manner he was from the upper crust, and she matched him with a strong and defiant rejoinder.

"Barry, James Miranda," she said, extending her gloved hand, "Pleased to make your acquaintance."

"Yes, yes the same for me," he said, again with a double tap. "The same for me. Now I must be off. I do so hope you have a pleasant day, despite the rawness of the weather. I dare say one's first day at Edinburgh can be quite memorable."

Pandora stopped a moment and watched him stride off self-assuredly toward the classrooms, glancing backwards at her once or twice. She thought it odd this lad had singled her out and as soon as there was some distance between them, she had the strange feeling that the mingling workmen and passing students were staring at her. But she gave no credence to these feelings because they derived, she assumed, from over sensitivity to her incognita.

"Ow!" she howled, flying forward and landing flat on her stomach. A young man tipped his hat to her as he sped by her. He had just kicked her squarely in the derriere. She jumped to her feet. But as the reproach was about to spring from her throat, another sharp thwank landed on her posterior and before she knew it she was again sprawled face down on the wet cobbles. Something fell over her head as she landed. Awkwardly she pulled it off her back, at the same time quickly getting to her feet in order to regain some dignity.

The object from her back was a sign which said in bright red letters:

PLEASE KICK MY ARSE
AS HARD AS YOU CAN

A pressure built in her temples as laughter cascaded down from a second story window packed with boys in the throes of an hysterical fit, jostling one another with exaggerated enthusiasm. Mr. Palmer stood in their midst looking down at her with a placid demeanor and supercilious grin. Slowly she turned and saw everywhere in the quadrangle, small groups of laughing young men who had obviously been watching the entire episode unfold. All were having a grand time at her expense.

With deliberate measure she ripped the sign again and again, but this only provoked applause and huzzahs from the crowd. She threw the little scraps into the air and prodded by her shame, took flight. Just then two burly workmen were rounding the corner carrying beer pails and wearing gaily colored hats. Reflexively she lifted her shoulders and buried her face, but she met them head on obstructing their path. She moved left, as did they, then with an awkward jerk she jumped right and to the roar of the attendant crowd, the two followed her lead. "Well, this is a lovely dance, lady, but we really must be back to work," said the one with the cocked tam-o'-shanter. Then both jumped aside and lifted their pails up over her head, forming an arch the way soldiers cross swords at a wedding. She flew underneath and ran through the quad out of the college proper.

She didn't stop until she found herself in the safety and seclusion of a partially demolished building. She pulled off her brand new surtout and holding it by one sleeve, she flayed the ground. The sounds of the laughter, the picture of their faces and the humiliation of those bruising kicks drove her deeper into a frenzy, torturing her, feeding her. She spun round and hurled the coat as hard as she could.

"Mr. Palmer indeed?" she spat. "Filthy bastard, have a nice day indeed, have a memorable day indeed!" She began to scream in French. "Filthy bastard, who the hell do they think they are, horrible filthy useless bastards?" Her fury blazed as she tore around the pit striking at anything within reach. Suddenly her shins struck hard an extended timber, toppling her over onto the filthy floor, whereupon she began beating at her legs with shocking malice, until her rage was spent. Her face soaked with tears, her nose an unchecked flow, she pulled her knees to her chest and sobbed quietly.

"I can't do it, it's too hard," she said,over and over. "I just don't have what it takes." Her despondency cloaked her with a terrible feeling of wretchedness, and she stayed drawn in that little knot for some time. After the sobs had ceased, she leaned back against the rubble with complete resignation and looked up at the dense gray sky through the wrenched timbers.

"My dearest General," she began. "Today I have decided not to become a doctor, not to heal the sick and not to be by your side as you build a democracy in Colombia. No, I am giving up totally any idea that such a magnificent dream could be aided by one as low and weak as I. As your humble servant I at least owe you an explanation for this sudden decision. I have given up my quest before having so much as taken one class at the university. In truth I have not even registered with the bursar. I have turned tail and run, noble General, thereby destroying any confidence you placed in me. I am, I see, a coward at heart, for I have allowed a pompous, ignorant, spoiled and stupid aristocratic hooligan to publicly abuse and humiliate me to such an extent that I am now hiding like a beaten dog. I regret for you, dear sir, that all of the faith you so generously awarded me was falsely seen and I believe now it would have been far better if you had left me to rot in the gutters of Paris, where you found me."

Something moved behind her. She turned.

There, poised atop a brick pedestal, one paw lifted and sniffing the air for her scent, was a sleek rat. Very slowly, with all the skill of her past, Pandora felt under the rubble for a small stone and whipping it in a quick silent shot, she knocked her prey off its perch, dead to the ground.

Even more than "L'homme de la boite," Pandora had hated these pediculous scavengers of the night, whose painful bites had marked every child who lived on the streets of Paris. She never missed a chance to lessen their number. It felt good to strike out at her old enemy.

Looking up at the sky again she saw instead of clouds the images of her youth. The men carrying buckets of blood from the guillotine to the Seine. A pretty young woman in a white dress with a blue ribbon entwined in her fingers, gently stroking the curly hair of her husband's disembodied head, as it lay in her blood soaked lap. She remembered the prisons and their smell, Haly and his vicious dog Ravage, how she had tamed them both to suit her purposes.

A sensation began to grow up her spine, making her skin tingle. "I walked in and out of every prison in Paris, for Christ's sake. I fought for my money with the toughest louts alive and wrested my daily bread however I could. I survived the goddamn French Revolution!" she exclaimed. "And now I'm being knocked off my course by nothing more than a little rat! Never!" She called out, "Never will I let this happen!"

She brushed off her pants and looked around for her discarded coat. If I am to be defeated, she thought, let it be from the rigors of my academic masters. She stood up, barely noticing the soreness of her bruised shins. Let defeat come from the strictures of time or the limits of my capacities, but not from garbage eating rats! Hurriedly she arranged herself and while she shook her surtout, she was flooded with renewed spirit. If they kick my bloody arse one hundred times a day, they will never drive me from my path, nor my precious obligation.

As she buttoned the last button on her coat, a new thought occurred to her. Actually, this entire event has been a very good sign. After all, it is not my intention to be taken for Sir Lancelot. Why, this humiliating situation has only confirmed for me my original consideration, that the success of the entire ruse lies in my being perceived as a small, studious and slightly eccentric fellow. The perfect target for boorish bullies. But, she continued feeling a good deal stronger, I did not realize that in the world of men and boys, such individuals as I are prey to so vile a scum as I have just encountered. I must resolve not to allow so base a person as Mr. Palmer to defeat me. I know why I am here and now I know what awaits me.

She was fully prepared to leave her hideout, yet she stopped for one last moment, her face becoming hardened, her eyes cold, "But," she said with callousness, "I will allow myself one luxury—revenge!"

Climbing over the wet stones and lumber awaiting their places in new buildings, Pandora calmly and confidently walked back toward her original destination.

***

The din in the bursar's office, which had been constant all morning, halted abruptly as soon as Pandora entered the room. With a defiant air she took her place in the line. Someone in the crowd shouted out, "Where's your sign, me boy? I hope you didn't lose it!" and the whole room, jammed with students, burst into spontaneous and raucous laughter.

The sharp voice of the bursar cut short the uproar. "I'll have order and decorum, gentlemen," he said, holding up his pince-nez for emphasis, "or by my word, none of you will be registered in the university this semester." The reluctant overseer was a bald-pated officious little man whose white cravat was so tightly tied round his starched collar it caused the blue veins of his neck to stand out right up to his temples. The herd of students obeyed his demand, though not without reluctance and a good deal of sniggering.

"One would think," said a round boy, loud enough for all ears, "that, at the very least, a brand new student would have some pride of dress. Didn't your Mummy teach you anything? Didn't she tell you one had to be neat and tidy their first day of school?" His voice came from directly behind Pandora. His remark provoked a low moan of appreciation from his clique. Encouraged, the fat boy continued. "Why, just look at you. Your coat's, dirty and disheveled, little curls a mess—and those knees! What could you *possibly* have been doing to have acquired such filthy, wet knees?"

Pandora saw him break into a wide grin of self-satisfaction. Facing him squarely she responded, "I appreciate your concern for my sartorial state and can assure you my mother's rearing was excellent. Then again, at least I know who mine was."

A low whistle went through the room as Pandora stood before her adversary, small and straight. "You see my friend, I had a strange accident this morning. But it was not totally without value, because it taught me an interesting lesson. I have learned that some of the men of Edinburgh appear to have more strength in their feet than they do in their heads. As a matter of fact it seems to me that someone such as yourself would be better equipped pursuing an education in blacksmithing, where your splendid bulk—obviously unencumbered by a brain—could be put to better use."

A round of applause and hoots went through the room. Pandora saw her interlocutor look around in disbelief, deeply wounded by the fickle sympathies of his supporters. Then with face beet red, he lunged at her, grabbing her by the lapels and lifting her off her feet. "I'll show you how smart you are, you miserable little bum sucker!"

"All right, that's enough now, let's put an end to it!" Pandora's knight was a dark haired, athletically built student with a square jaw. He separated the two combatants with clear authority. The fat boy immediately took a step back. Pandora could see from the look on his face that he was not about to challenge this tall, strapping lad.

"We'll take this matter up again at another time," he said, and stormed out through the jeers of the crowd.

"I'm John Jobson, pleased to make your acquaintance Mr—?"

"Barry," Pandora said, shaking his hand enthusiastically. "James Barry."

CHAPTER TWENTY-FOUR

"Chemistry, my fine and bright-eyed gentlemen, is not nearly as young as many of you may think. No, she is as old a dame as any other science, yet she still holds youth in her look and vigor springs her gait."

Sitting in the rear of the lecture hall, poised like an arrow pulled back in its bow, Pandora followed every movement the black-cloaked professor made, as he gracefully stalked like a Bengal tiger, in and out among the glass apparatus he used for the demonstration of this wondrous science. "Whenever man begins to speculate on the inner constitution of matter, he becomes a chemist."

Pandora could not write fast enough to keep pace. Her head bobbed up and down from paper to professor in a vainglorious attempt to capture it all. "Therefore," he continued, "when Aristotle said that matter is composed of earth, fire, water and air—he was not speaking as a philosopher—but as a chemist." Pandora's heart beat loudly in her ear as she bore down on her pencil, while these ideas reached into her head like two powerful hands, and turned her mind.

Expecting to share her excitement with her fellow classmates, she looked around the worn amphitheater. In place of eagerness, the first thing which met her eye was the sight of a sleeping boy hiding behind his propped up book, ash blond hair flopped over his brow. Then across the way she spotted a diminutive lad, straining forward on the bench, his elfin face wrinkled with perplexity. Jesus and Mary! she thought as she moved from face to face, I don't believe it! They really don't get it. What's the matter with them? Don't they have ears? Aren't his words ringing in their heads? She felt like standing up and scolding the lot of them.

"The old boy's playing with a hot hand today," whispered her friend John Jobson, never once looking up from his note-taking. He was the son of a Scottish country doctor and had quickly grasped the principles of chemistry. He already attained the position of vice-president of the chemistry club.

"Nothing but trumps," she shot back out of the corner of her mouth.

"Gentlemen," said Professor Hope, "I must warn you that the Almighty, in his infinite wisdom, pressed me from the exact same mold as my illustrious predecessor, Dr. Boyle. I, too, am a skeptical chemist who believes in the experiment with the same fervor as did Moses in the word of God." Delighted at his apt comparison, Dr. Hope allowed himself a broad smile then continued. "Boyle said, 'Methinks the chemists, in their search after truth are not unlike the navigators of Solomon's fleet who brought home from their long and tedious voyages, not only gold, silver and ivory, but apes and peacocks too.' So today, fellow sailors, our journey will course through the treacherous straits of combustion—and God only knows what we will find there. For no problem has been so important nor incessant in its plaguing as our difficulty in understanding the process of combustion and the mystery of flame.

"The very first secret man had to wrest from God was the trick of making fire. He needed it to warm his body, to protect him while he slept and to entertain his mind as he sat on the empty plains in front of its glow, eons before the record of history." Dr. Hope spread his arms wide embracing his audience. "Prometheus lighted his torch on the wheel of the sun. And the ascension of man had begun. For a short time after we were satisfied. We roasted our game, illuminated our caves and mumbled pious thanks.

"But it is not in the nature of our species to remain content for long. Our greed rose. It was not enough for us to call forth flame at will. Oh, no! We wanted still more, a peek under the skirts of the burning embers, to see the very stuff of which the fire mistress was made."

Dr. Hope filled the pause with piercing scrutiny. Pandora imagined he knew those students who understood and those who did not. "This proved to be a quixotic problem indeed, wooing the best minds of science for the last two thousand years."

He now positioned himself in the center of the stage before them, "It was believed that the secret of fire had something to do with the observable fact that when bodies were burned, something escaped. This something came to be called, in relatively modern time, phlogistin, so uncovered and named by a physician to the King of Prussia, Herr George Ernst Stahl. This man believed that combustible objects were rich in this phlogistin, and when burning took place, the element was lost, leaving behind matter devoid of it.

"Thus, lads, the ash in your fireplace is wood with all the phlogistin spent. Most of us fully accepted Herr Stahl's doctrine, until one day, less than forty years ago, an English chemist named Joseph Priestley, while on a tour of France, discussed his recent experiments in the making of dephlogisticated-air with a group of scientists at the Paris home of M. Antoine Laurant Lavoisier."

A glimmer of recognition shot through Pandora as she stopped her note taking. She remembered the lovely day in May, when she had arrived at the prison to find it heavy with sadness—every one of her "professors" highly agitated and capable only of talking about the unpardonable beheading of this already great man. "M. Lavoisier," Dr. Hope's high-toned voice broke in, scattering her recollection, "having long been fascinated with the whole question of combustion, incorporated the Englishman's experiments into his own work. He went on to overthrow the doctrine of phlogistin, thereby thrusting us into the modem age of chemistry.

"Only he understood that what Priestley had isolated was not air without phlogistin, but another element entirely. It was, as he said, 'the purest portion of the air, more respirable, and more combustible.' He came to call it oxygen."

Dr. Hope stepped forward now, raising his head to address the gallery. "And what was the world's response to having such a man in its midst? Logically, one would assume the highest honors would be bestowed upon him. Everything essential for his workplace put at his disposal."

Stepping up onto the front rung of the amphitheater, Hope slapped his thigh for emphasis. "That is what a logical man would assume. But, while the affairs of the universe conform to pristine formulae, alas, the affairs of man do not. So, with an ignorance typical of our kind," he said, charging up the steps, voice ringing round the room, "Antoine Laurant Lavoisier was taken from his laboratory one bloody spring and placed upon the guillotine—the secrets of nature nevermore to unveil."

He had come to rest on the step right next to the enthralled Pandora, who try as she might, could not look up to his face. So overwhelmed was she by his proximity.

"A fellow scientist said when hearing of Lavoisier's execution, 'A moment was all that was necessary to strike off his head and probably one hundred years will not be sufficient to produce another one like it.'"

The lecture hall was silent, while Professor Hope presiding from atop the stairs, looked down at the pit below. One by one the rest of the class followed his lead and for a flash of time, it seemed as if the ghost of M. Lavoisier himself was down there, roaming among the beakers and tall jars, conjured to this hallowed chamber of science, by the exalted words of their tutor.

What a miraculous teacher he is, Pandora thought. She could not believe the change which had taken place in the room. Now all, save the somnambulist boy, were charged with life, their faces keen with wonder. She wanted to look up at this great man, but now she was afraid if she did his steely blue eyes would penetrate hers and he would discover the secret through her transpicuous disguise. Then what would he do? In her mind's eye, she saw him lifting her up by the collar, "Well what do we have here, me ladies? An impostor in our very midst, not a fine fellow like the rest of you, but a deceiver, a fraud, a pretender of the highest order. Out! Get out! There's no place for the likes of you here!"

"Well, that's enough morbidity for one afternoon," announced Professor Hope, bringing her back with a start. "After all, this is a chemistry class, not Mr. Fyfe's dissecting morgue, and I assume everyone in here is still among the living." The professor marched down the stops and hard knuckled the head of the sleeping blond boy as he passed.

"All right, Ma, I'm up," he groaned with filial consternation, and the room fell into hearty laughter. Pandora looked at Jobson and they too joined in.

"I'm all right, Ma, I'm up!" she chortled to herself, but something in the ludicrousness of the boy's remark struck a deep chord, releasing her girlish laugh, which spread out quickly around her. Feeding on itself, her abandon built until she was swaying back and forth and side to side.

The blond boy wheeled round, "What's so funny, nan-boy!" he shouted up at her.

"All right Ma, I'm up!" she squeezed out again. Her contageous laughter started an epidemic which leapfrogged from row to row. Driven by his humiliation, the boy picked up his book, which moments ago had served as his shield, and prepared to heave it at her. When he stepped back, his foot slipped, sending him bouncing from chair to floor with a great clattering noise. Pandora squealed again.

Everyone, including Dr. Hope, was defenseless in the face of her musical hurrah. Each time a fresh seizure shook her, they all echoed back in kind. Finally, Professor Hope called for order by rapping the slate table with a metal rule.

"That'll do, lads, that'll do! Now if the masters of the chemistry club will regain their composure, and please come to my assistance, we shall proceed with today's experiment."

John Jobson rose and so did Mr. Smythe, who had been sitting down front. "This is a fine one, James," Jobson said, and bounded down the stairs.

"The loftiness of science," continued Dr. Hope, "rests firmly on the shoulders of demonstrable proof, not on the gossamer wings of fanciful conjecture." Mr. Jobson and Mr. Smythe cleared the decks while Mr. Davidson, the lab assistant, wheeled over the star of the experiment, a large, lidded glass jar filled with oxygen.

Pandora began to diagram the experiment with single-minded concentration. Suddenly there was the sound of much bustle, as the three leaders of the Ten Drink Club took up positions in the row behind her. "Now, boys!" whispered Penwell Palmer, their president. "I'm going to show you an exceptional experiment of my own. I do believe," he pressed, "if I were to strike the back of Barry's head with the proper implement, I would be able to produce the most rounded and rich tones anyone has ever heard."

"Les eretins horreurs ont arrivé!" she mumbled with disgust, as she moved forward on the bench creating as much distance as possible between herself and them. "Well, what will you hit the bell with, Penny," the fat boy chirped in on cue. "A small hammer would be the perfect thing," Penwell whispered into Pandora's ear. "Perhaps you have in your possession such an implement, Mr. Barry. I've heard you are quite well-equipped."

As the three boys laughed, Pandora sat like stone, praying that Dr. Hope would commence the experiment, which would return his attention to the room thus impeding her tormentors.

"Why, Mr. Barry," said Penwell, "it's not very social of you to ignore us in such a cold fashion. I realize, of course, our friendship has not gotten off on the surest of footings, but I cannot understand your reluctance to remedy the situation with a simple response. After all, aren't you interested in science? Aren't you just the least bit curious to know what sound your head will make when struck with the appropriate instrument?"

"I don't have a hammer, Penny, but I think this will do." Pandora recognized the pinched voice of Mr. Beaufort. She wanted nothing more than to turn round and see what that horrid acne-ridden larrikin had come up with. But she knew she couldn't because if she showed them the slightest sign of fear, it was certain she would never have another moment's peace.

"A clay pipe, Mr. Beaufort? Very ingenious! May I speak to you plainly, Mr. Barry?" Penwell asked as he tapped the weapon against his palm. "After all, we have so much in common you and I, that I feel there should be no artificial barriers between us. So you must understand, it is not without great pain, that I tell you of my deep disappointment in your character. We all had such high hopes for you. Why, we even entertained the notion that one day you might join our little club. But now, when your assistance is so vitally needed in order to accomplish an important academic endeavor, what do you do, my cox-combed friend—?" Penwell paused, cocking back the clay pipe, "—you turn to us with a deaf ear!" He cracked Pandora a crisp rap, hitting the bone behind her ear. "There, gentlemen!" he said with a victorious air. "Proof positive, the head is hollow!"

The sting bit deep, a charge of pain shot through her and the sensitive flesh throbbed and began to trickle blood. Pandora fought back her hand, which wanted to give comfort. With all her resolve she refused to move a muscle, keeping her eyes fixed on the apparatus being assembled.

"Gentlemen," Dr. Hope said addressing his helpers, "would you please bring over, with care, the charcoal brazier?" Mr. Jobson and Mr. Smythe donned heavy gloves and lifted the metal box containing the glowing embers, across the floor to the place indicated.

Emboldened by Penwell's success, the sharp-nosed Beaufort tapped Pandora on the shoulder. "Please sir," he asked, "may I borrow a sheet of your paper?" Then without a moment's hesitation, he ripped her carefully drawn diagram from its binding. "Thank you very much!" he snorted, throwing himself back onto the bench while tearing it to tatters. The other two boys pulled her back by the shoulders and Beaufort stuffed the scraps down her shirt.

"Mr. Barry," added the fat one, "we're so happy you decided to study at Edinburgh. Why, whatever would we have done without you!"

CHAPTER TWENTY-FIVE

"James," John Jobson asked with a tentative tongue, as the two friends walked through the Kings Park, shrouded in the thick morning fog. "I have to ask you something straight out and forward." They had come to their favorite hill which met up with the bridle path, and as usual at this hour, there was no evidence that any of the gaily dressed riders who frequented these environs had yet arrived.

"Well go ahead, John, ask away," Pandora said, as they stepped onto the cinders and commenced up the incline.

"I know I can count on you to answer me honestly." Jobson stopped, allowing Pandora to gain on him. She turned when she realized she was walking alone. "James?" Jobson said. "Are you a queer?"

"A what?" she shot back, dumbstruck.

"You know, a queer. A rum, a nan-boy—a fellow who fancies other fellows."

"I don't have any idea what you're talking about," she said, stalling in order to construct her answer.

"Please, James," Jobson said, drawing lines onto the cinder path with his boot. "I know this is ugly business, so the sooner we rid ourselves of it the better. Do you prefer kissing lads or lassies?" The fog rolled around the two darkly-clad figures. Pandora felt strangely calm, watching her friend's discomfort. Surprisingly, she found that she was not in the least concerned at the possible threat to her discovery.

"As busy as I've been with my own studies and trying to push some Latin through that astoundingly thick skull of yours, I dare say whatever my predilection, I've had scant enough time to execute it. But, in response to your first inquiry, as to whether or not I am, as you say, a 'queer', let me assure you, my good friend, that my kissing desires are identical and in conformity to all those of my sex."

"Good!" said Jobson, his entire body emphasizing his disburdenment.

"Your relief suggests you had doubts."

"I am not trying to suggest anything. As you know I have no desire to hurt you in any way. But there are some ugly rumors which surround your person. Let's face it, you're not the most common fellow."

This elicited from Pandora her high pitched laugh, which shook her shoulders.

"There," said Jobson, "that's exactly what I mean! If you'd change that laugh of yours, maybe you could dampen the swirl of malicious gossip that goes around about the very matter I just broached and—"

"Commenced and perpetuated no doubt," Pandora interrupted, "by Mr. Robin Penwell Palmer and his colleagues. Am I correct?"

"Just so, James. But I must add here that you have not helped dispel any of their malevolent behavior toward you."

"I don't understand you, John."

The two companions had finally reached the top of the knoll and were looking down into the small mist covered valley which separated them from the university and those of whom they spoke. "Penwell and the rest put you at their mercy with their heinous pranks the minute I turn my back, only because you refuse to produce any sign of manly challenge. They will only continue to humiliate you and spread their horrid rumors, unless you yourself strike a clear blow of retaliation."

"I'm sorry, John, it is impossible. I am not that sort of person. I'm not good at the rough stuff."

"You're not afraid, are you? Why, that Beaufort is not much bigger than you and with a few pugilistic lessons from me, you could probably present a good showing. The important thing here, James, is that whatever the outcome, your actions will put these stories to rest."

"No, John, I am afraid they wouldn't. But I am no coward and

I mean to defeat those rascals, not merely hush unchecked gossip. My uncommonness calls for another method of victory, not some inept show of bravado. No, I must defeat Robin Penwell Palmer and his gang with the strength of my brain!"

"Honestly, James, sometimes I think you live in another world entirely. People like this will not be defeated by some clever notion dreamt up in that facile brain of yours. No, these are matters that call for fists, not fantasies. And I'll be damned if I don't think that you deliberately encourage them to view you this way."

"Well, Mr. Jobson," Pandora rebutted. "I realize my peculiarities make it difficult for me and those who find themselves in my association. And I understand that there will be times when it would be easier to sever such an uncomfortable alliance. So if you wish to withdraw from our friendship, I want you to know—I think you are a coward who's knuckling under the weight of social pressure propagated by a bunch of small-minded fops." She started to walk away.

"Now calm yourself man," Jobson said, catching up and putting his arm around her shoulders, "I just needed to get on the straight line. Besides," he said, allowing some laughter to ease their moods, "how else will I ever learn the Latin I need to defend my thesis? I'm glad the air is cleared. And James, you know with only one word from you, I'd teach Mr. Palmer a lesson he'll not soon forget."

They had come across the crags, the cold drizzle tapped their hats.

"No, John," Pandora said, "your intervention would only make matters worse and stimulate the flap of their filthy tongues. I have another plan, which this morning's outing has nurtured. Let us go and see Mr. Davidson at the chemistry lab. I think between the three of us, we can make it work."

CHAPTER TWENTY-SIX

"It's simply incredible!" rose the pompous twang of Robin Penwell Palmer's voice, above the din in the packed pub. "She doesn't look any older? Does she, lads?" The barmaid's young spherical face was flushed red as she made effort to refill their empty pints. "And this is no small feat, for it seems it's been near a decade since last we placed our orders."

"I am sorry, sir!" the buxom girl begged, "but as you can plainly see, we're a fright busy! And two of us is out sick."

"Out sick, are you?" scorned Penwell, holding the full attention of his crammed table. "My dear girl!" he spoke not as much to her as to his appreciative fellows, "the health and well being of the servant-girl population in the city of Edinburgh is not the slightest concern to me. No, mademoiselle, my concern is the swiftness of service, which I and my constituents, of the Ten Drink Club, receive!"

"Hear, hear!" cheered several of the boys sitting around the table, which was littered with the debris of many rounds and the soot of careless smokers. "In fact if—," Penwell grabbed hold of the departing girl's tray, bullying her further, " —if such lackadaisical service becomes habitual, I will have to use my not inconsiderable influence with the management to make sure someone with more efficiency is engaged!"

The girl, who looked to be barely fifteen, freed her salver and hastily pushed her way through the crush of young men who always jammed the back room of the Ten Drink Pub.

James Barry and John Jobson were standing not far from the table watching, as she squeezed by, balancing her overload with remarkable dexterity. Mr. Beaufort, who had followed her departure with a lascivious eye, spotted the two and sprayed the ale he just swigged all over the table. "Look there," he choked out, elbowing Penwell, then pointing at the silent observers.

"My, my, my!" Penwell said rising to his feet with semi-inebriated grandeur. "If it isn't the unsociable Mr. Barry, and his dear, dear friend, Mr. Jobson. Boys, on your feet! Make way and move over, for our surprise guests!"

Their mien giving away no secrets, John Jobson and Pandora took the chairs proffered them. Pandora, stiff backed and full of confidence took the one next to Mr. Penwell, while Jobson sat on her left.

"Mr. Barry, whatever could it be that brings you out on this winter's night? To what do we owe the pleasure of so surprising a visit?" Penwell turned to face Jobson, pointing his glass toward him, "Your friend Jobson has been here on several occasions, but until now, it seems he has been unable to convince you to accompany him and partake in the conviviality of your fellow classmen."

Pandora sensed the crowd filling in behind her, but she held steady, her eye on Robin. "I had a taste and mind for sport, so I thought I'd search you out," she said.

"Well," Penwell scoffed, draining his dram. "What is so special about me?" He reclaimed his seat now and those nearby pressed closer to hear the little redhead's response.

"I thought you might provide me with an evenings entertainment, as I have heard *rumor* – " She leaned on the word. " – that you are a chap who really holds his liquor and rare is the fellow who can match you in that heroic and manly art."

"What's your proposition?" Penwell asked. Pandora played the crowd, by waiting in silence. Then Jobson rose and tossed his money pouch on the table.

"A drinking bout, until one man drops!" he said. "Five pounds to the winner, loser pays for the spirits." The grin that spread across Penwell's face was far from sober and Pandora noted his glassy eyes.

"Perhaps," she said, "we ought to do this some other day. Since it appears you have already had a few, and as I haven't yet begun, it would put you at a disadvantage."

Beaufort and the rotund Reginald roared.

"On the contrary, Mr. Barry, I've only just wet my whistle. And I fear if I allow you to slip into the night, I will forever have lost this golden opportunity! Reginald!" he snapped. "Do you have five pounds,"

"No, Penny," Reginald whined, "but I have two." As Reginald searched his tight pockets for the two pounder. There rose from all around them the sound of loose change and spirited shouts. "Two Pence," "I've got a quid!" Penwell smiled as the ante built up.

"You're on!" he said, patting the funds piling up center table.

"Splendid!" Pandora said, a serene smile matching his arrogant one.

"Well then," Penwell said, the grin still stuck on his face. "How many do we start with and what is your fare?"

"I see you are drinking brandy, Mr. Palmer. This is most fortunate, for it seems we have this in common. It is my one weakness," Barry confided to the crowd. "Let's make it ten for starters!"

"Barmaid!" shouted Jobson, "two bottles of the best, and twenty glasses!" By now as many as could, crammed the back room of the pub. Those who couldn't get in climbed the tables and banquettes, to have a look at the action from over the glass partitions, which separated one room from the other. Everyone held a glass or pint, and reports of the proceedings were relayed as they occurred, followed by a lot of commentary, and spiced with rigorous side-betting.

Barry straight-lined the ten glasses, brought by the stout barmaid. "Would you please sit next to me, my dear? I know that you will bring me luck," she said to the harried serving girl, who was not quite certain what to do. But when Jobson relinquished his chair to her, she smiled and sat.

"One thing gentlemen," Jobson said, filling each of Barry's glasses. "Mr. Barry prefers a cognac flambé, if that is acceptable with all,"

"What on earth is a cognac flambé?" groused Beaufort.

"Never mind!" Penwell stopped him. "That's fine by me, John. Whatever the little fellow wants to make it easier is just fine."

Pandora remained in her perfect state of calm allowing, nothing to ruffle her. "Miss," Jobson said, handing a lit wick to the barmaid, "would you do us the honor and touch a flame to each glass?"

One after the other, a blue flame appeared and danced on the brandy. When the first one flickered out Pandora lifted her glass and delicately drained it. Palmer shot back his first five in quick succession. The crowd urged him on, then grew silent as they watched Barry methodically continue, drink by drink, just as the moment each flame died away.

"Mr. Penwell," Barry said, when she had caught up with Robin. "Are you still sure you wish to continue? Your color, my man, does not bode well."

"You are obviously not seeing too well, Mr. Barry," Mr. Palmer said, downing three more and beginning to sweat on his upper lip. "You're behind. I've only got two more to go.

Pandora kept her eyes on the now ghastly pale fellow, as she ever more gracefully downed her next three. Then Penwell effortfully finished nine, and slowly, as if he were raising lead, brought the last to his lips. From the way he pursed them, Pandora saw, he was losing control and from the slight jerk of his shoulders, she knew he was holding down the contents of his stomach, with much difficulty.

"Mr. Barry?" Jobson said, indicating his last two, their flames dying. Pandora swallowed one quickly, to a mild cheer. Then with a flourish, she daintily polished off the last. "The first round is done!" cried Jobson, his words repeated throughout, for the far room. "Ten more glasses please!" Two trays, already set up, floated toward them from hand to hand, accompanied by shouts.

"Yes, ten more, excellent, very good," slurred Mr. Palmer as he struggled to his feet. "A perfectly excellent idea. But first I must—!" Suddenly Robin Penwell Palmer retched violently, spewing forth the night's drinking onto the waistcoat of his second, Mr. Beaufort, whose admiring grin vanished with the shock. Then he fell to the floor in a groaning mess.

"Such uncouth behavior for a well-bred gentleman," Pandora said to the barmaid, whose sweet face glowed with delight as the members of the Ten Drink Club attempted to prop their champion onto his chair.

"Is your man ready to continue?" Jobson asked, in a totally unconcerned manner.

"I'MMMM–SWELL!" forced Penwell, his jaw hanging agape, his mess staining his moleskin breeches. Jobson completed the line of glasses and was about to light them, when the smell from the liquor struck Penwell's nose and he heaved afresh. He vainly tried to arrest the loss of all dignity with his handkerchief, but, done in, he meekly waved the unserviceable bib in surrender. The mob sent up a wild cheer and those nearby slapped the victorious Barry on the back and tousled her bright red hair.

"Thank you for being good-luck." Barry leaned into the startled barmaid, while he caught Jobson's wink from the next seat.

"But, you're so little a fellow!" the awed girl said. "How in the name of the Lord Jesus did you drink so much alcohol?" Her question could be heard in repetition through the room.

Then James Barry rose, stood on the chair she had occupied, and triumphantly addressed the good-willed throng. "The answer is simple, my friends. I can't drink so much alcohol, and I didn't. As any good chemistry student knows–alcohol burns!"

At first all remained quiet, letting the words sink in. Then slowly as recognition deepened, a chant began, "Alcohol Bums! Alcohol Burns!" Two stalwart youths picked up Pandora, chair and all, while the chant built. The students danced round the pub then out into the night with their hero, heralding the cry, "Alcohol Burns! Alcohol Burns!"

CHAPTER TWENTY-SEVEN

The glare of the high sun made Pandora squint as she rushed down the little path towards the old surgeons' hall. Barely acknowledging the shouts of greeting friends, she pressed on to the entryway of number nine, a small detached house next door to the main hall. She banged the door behind and then grabbed her breath, before walking through the anatomy hall to the narrow stair which descended under the demonstration arena to the dissecting room below. There was an acrid bite to the cold draft which assaulted her as she started down to the windowless "Dead House," and the "good old surgical stink" as always took a bit of getting used to. Her eyes watered and she breathed carefully until she landed at the bottom and could resume a normal intake. Nose and eyes acclimated themselves to both the fetid air and the candle light.

"Ah, Mr. Barry! My day is now complete," said Mr. Fyfe, moving away from the two students he was assisting. "Quickly, son, make yourself ready for work."

Pandora nodded toward the two dissectionists who smiled a brief hello, then returned to their cadaver—a bearded young man who lay flat, head propped-up, staring at his feet. His fore skull had been removed, exposing his brain, which they probed and prodded. At another table, stretched supine, rested a woman's body whose demise was attributable to her love of gin. Her face was bloated and the blotches, akin to alcoholism had turned an eerie purplish-blue. The novices working over her were removing her cataract eye, which wore a sharp white spot.

"I have a real prize for you today," Fyfe said, abandoning the first pair, his candle dripping wax over his hands while the plaited wick burned smoky. "I've found you the perfect inguinal hernia." Fyfe winked, taking his favorite student round the shoulders. "They're much better to work on after they've passed from a long and lingering disease," he said, leading her to table number three. "It displays the groin area much more clearly."

Pandora saw the body laid out under a cloth, a disposal tub positioned under the table, instruments already resting on the covered belly.

"I sent for you as soon as he came in." Fyfe lifted the instruments and thrust back the sheet. "Over here, lads! Let's lift him up. One of you gentlemen bring me the wood blocks." Pandora had rolled up her sleeves, and approached the skeletal old fellow, while Fyfe placed the wood blocks onto the table. "Now lay him down right here," he said to the two, adjusting the blocks under the cadaver's loins.

"Fine, fine, exactly in place. Let me slip this leg over the side and that'll give us a solid look at the situation. James, get in close. After all, this is your winning today."

The boys with the red-headed woman stopped their ocular exploration and joined the others in order to receive instruction from the master dissector. "Eh, eh, eh," Fyfe said, stepping back, indicating to Pandora to take up the tools. "Direct inguinal strangulation. Would you please proceed Mr. Barry?"

Pandora moved in, first spreading the tools between the corpse's legs, then gently she probed the groin area. She was pleased with how clearly defined the tumor was and wasted no time making the first vertical incision, from just under the umbelicus, clear and straight, to the front of the scrotum.

"Good, son," Fyfe encouraged, his pigtail dancing up and down as he nodded. "Now the second."

She continued steadily down and across making a perfect triangular flap, exposing the fascia superficialis.

"Excellent, James." Fyfe tapped the table lightly. "Now let us dissect the fascia superficialis, from the tendon of the external oblique."

Swiftly and surely Pandora moved her scalpel along. She felt her own confidence and excitement gaining, yet she didn't allow the slightest waver in her scissions.

"Notice there is a very slight attachment to the tendon and see there, lads, the connection between the spermatic chord is as inconsiderable. James," he said, "the handle of your knife should push down all the way between the chord and tendon, as far down as to the bottom of the scrotum."

Pandora's delicate hands gently forced the handle, separating the tissue just as Mr. Fyfe had directed. Pride flooded through her as she proceeded. "We must remove all loose fat from the lower part of the chord," Fyfe instructed, handing her forceps and scissors. She began to work with an increasing pace, prompted by her own inner rhythm. She loved the exactness and dare each step demanded.

"Now," Fyfe said, halting her and giving her one of those smiles reserved for a prized pupil, "let's cut the tendon of the external oblique, in two directions. From the superior anterior spinous process of the ilium, to the linea alba, and the other from the linea alba to the pubis." The students rearranged themselves around the table to better see Barry execute the procedure.

"Be careful when you separate the extended oblique from the internal oblique," cautioned Fyfe. Pandora leaned into the body continuing to cut. "Good, that's fine, now fasten the muscle to the forepart of the thigh." She took a small hook from the edge of the table and pulling the loose muscle tissue back, she pressed the hook hard into the bony leg.

"Now, gentlemen," Fyfe announced, "as you can see, we have a perfect view of the inguinal canal." The four young men all leaned over the body and peered avidly inside. "Mr. Brown?" Fyfe said, invitingly. "Would you tell us the difference between what is muscle and what is chord?"

Mr. Brown looked quite some time. He even probed with his fingers, but the look of consternation that finally washed over his face made it unquestionable that he was stuck.

"It's the cremaster muscle that's confusing you," Pandora said with reassuring consideration, not intending arrogance. "If you pull the chord in the direction of the scrotum, you'll see the internal oblique is not attached to the whole extent of the Pouparts ligament, and see here," she said, reaching into the cavity, "the chord passes under the internal oblique, not through it!"

The satisfaction she felt from her own explanation made her a little breathless, and Mr. Fyfe's approving grin brought a slight flush to her cheeks. "All right let us now trace the course of the hernia to the scrotum," Fyfe said, taking up a scalpel and moving into Pandora's place. "Let us see what was the probable cause of stricture," Mr. Fyfe began, his shoulders rounded in a soft curve. He reminded Pandora of her old teacher Mr. Barry, when he would labor on one of his canvases.

* * *

The Examination Hall
Edinburgh University

"Gentlemen," Dr. Munro said. "Our next candidate is Mr. James Barry."

The extremity of Pandora's tension made her want to look only at the ground. But she fought against it, and as resolutely as possible. She held her head up and faced her six black-robed examiners squarely. They were all seated around a long table placed on the platform in front of the hall, and in defiance of her nerves, she took a moment to look at each one of them.

"Mr. Barry's doctoral thesis," Munro said, "is entitled 'De Merocele Vel Hernia Crurali.'"

The five other professors nodded acknowledgment and scrutinized the candidate while Dr. Munro opened the cover page of Pandora's meticulously penned document.

"Mr. Barry, I see here in the front piece of your thesis a quotation from Menander the Greek. 'Do not consider my youth, but consider instead whether or not I show the wisdom of a man?'"

"Sir?" Dr. Munro leaned forward and smiled warmly. "In the past days you have fulfilled the two prerequisite parts of your final examination and are about to defend, in Latin, your thesis on hernias of the groin. Let me assure you that the only criteria by which you will be judged is the degree to which you succeed in these tasks." He leaned back against the dark frame of his chair and folded his hands in his lap.

Perspiration nestled in the palms of Pandora's hands. She squeezed them tight behind her to steady her nerves. But the horrible fear that she had forgotten all she had learned took hold of her, and she imagined when she opened her mouth nothing would come out and she would leave the room in disgrace, all of her efforts having been for naught.

"The satisfactory accomplishment of these three formidable proceedings," Dr. Munro continued, "will determine whether or not you are to be granted a degree from this university. If so affirmed, you will be awarded the rights and privileges commensurate with the title, Doctor of Medicine."

Doctor of Medicine—the words breathed pure oxygen onto the fire within her, scorching the fear. Suddenly she was in the midst of a whirlwind of images: sitting untiringly beside a frail, despaired-of old man to ease him through his final moments, cradling a wet and wailing newborn in her arms, and probing with new and intricate instruments the mysterious organs of the human body. These were the things that had kept her here at Edinburgh, had driven her with ever vigorous passion from the lecture halls, to the clinics, to the dissecting room.

Initially, her love for and devotion to General Miranda had been her spark, but now the fire roared through the aegis of a different source. Somewhere in these last years she had discovered her purpose, the sole reason for which she was born and as she stood before these learned men, she had no doubt as to what this purpose was, Doctor of Medicine. It was now only a hair's breadth away and nothing was going to stop her.

"In a direct inguinal hernia," challenged Dr. Munro, "what is the frequency and cause of the spermatic chord being anterior to the hernial sac?"

As the Latin began to roll from her lips, she was imbued with the confidence, surety and the calm that comes from knowing. As her explanation proceeded she felt more like a colleague than a student. The deep mysteries she explained and the miracle of cure she promised thrilled her and she could see on her examiners' faces that they were proud of their university, their profession and of her.

Part II

CHAPTER ONE

"Though I write to you locked in the bowels of a Spanish prison," Sarah read, with a tremulous voice, "both my spirit and unwavering hope for a glorious future remain high."

The words had cast a heavy pall in the library at Grafton Street. The warm candle glow and all the familial faces gathered round the long table could not ease Sarah's struggle with her obstinate tears. At last she gave way and put the letter down. Pandora reached over and gently picked it up.

"As you can well imagine," she read, "when I received word from you of Pandora's recent historic accomplishment, I wished to run around this dark, dank cell, shouting her praises and laughing with joy for all to hear. But, alas, I am quite set apart from others, so my elation could only be shared with the unseen creatures who dwell behind stones or down small holes in my floor, and the private pictures of you all which I carry in my heart. My greatest deprivation now is being so far from you at this time, when there is so much triumph to share.

"Leander, my son, your promotion to the rank of captain gives me great pride."

Pandora looked over at Leander sitting in his father's chair. He filled it well, his back soldierly straight despite the sling he wore on his right arm and the heavy bandages around his protruding hand. His countenance bespoke a new maturity, not just in his handsomely sculpted features but in something that emanated from his dark, brooding eyes and overall composure.

"It is your valor and courage on the battlefield that have moved my hardened old soldier's soul to deep sentiment. Your wound, though I understand it to be quite painful, I am sure will soon be healed and will become nothing more than a proud badge of a distinguished soldier. Both of you, Pandora and Leander, have been brave and broad-shouldered, and I speak with the utmost confidence when I say that even though the prize of my mission has slipped through my fingers, it is not lost forever, and I trust in God that it will bring you both to me very soon."

Topham twirled his cap round and round in his big hands, his head hung below his hunched shoulders. Carmen and Rosa stood in the doorway, their fingers knitted together. Sarah remained as she had all along, full of sadness.

"I beseech you all not to despair for me, for despair is a malady of such lethal infectiousness that once it takes hold its progress is nearly impossible to stanch. I close with my deepest love, esteem, and congratulations to you all. Your devoted servant, General Francisco de Miranda."

"It's six months old," Sarah said, while Pandora folded the well worn paper. "It's difficult to smuggle out word, they watch him so closely. God only knows where they'll move him next. There's rumor of Cadiz." Sarah fought valiantly but could hold back the blackness no more.

Pandora could not believe what had happened to this woman of perpetual beauty. She had lost the radiance in her eyes to sadness; her remarkable skin, despite a careful rouging, showed only pallor, and her heretofore lush and vibrant mane was pulled tight and sternly from her too thin face. She was already a woman in mourning, convinced she had lost her love forever. Everyone was drawn to her pain and, fearing she was right, they were afraid to look at her.

"Mother..." Leander rose and stood behind Sarah, putting his good hand firmly on her shoulder. "I believe Father would be terribly disappointed in us if he could see how we were languishing about in all this gloom and doom. I'm certain our forces will rally in due time, if they have not already, and very soon we will see the general again."

Pandora was moved by Leander's mastery of the situation, so like General Miranda he was after all, the consummate male, the self-assured warrior in whom one immediately placed one's faith.

"And if, God forbid, this is the end...," Leander took his mother's hand, "...we will face it with the same courage he does."

Pandora saw that Sarah accepted Leander's words.

"We must remember that this is the life he chose to live," Leander said, to his father's friend Lord Buchan, "and that he lived it with a fullness and sincerity equaled by no man."

"Here, here," said Lord Buchan.

"Amen." Topham's voice was hoarse.

And Carmen in her usual way pressed down her apron and left the room.

"Lord Buchan, would you be so kind and provide us a toast to Pandora and General Miranda," Leander said, bringing the decanter to him.

Could it be, thought Pandora, that this was Leander's way of saying all was forgiven, and that as head of the household he had accepted all she had chosen?

CHAPTER TWO

Pandora slipped under the coolness of her sheets, comforted by the familiarity of her room above the library, which Sarah had kept just the way she had left it. Barely able to finish one page of her book, she blew out her candle and drifted off to sleep.

She found herself a child again, passing as a ghost through thick slime-soaked stone walls, entering and leaving one pitch black chamber after another. What prison this was she did not know, but she knew she was searching for General Miranda, and each time she heard a moan or a chain rattle, she hesitated and whispered his name. Suddenly, she heard someone singing a Spanish tune. She peered toward the form chained to the wall. It was unmistakably his strong voice but his body was covered with terrible red welts under shredded clothing. She saw large black blotches of dry blood across his chest and shoulders and his hair was a tangled mat of knots falling into his swollen eyes. "General Miranda," she said.

"Dear child," he said, his voice strong, full of verve. "You've come at last. I knew you wouldn't fail me." He smiled and tried to rise and go toward her, but his chain pulled him back down.

She reached out and was about to touch his hand when a great cracking sound burst the air. A wall behind her fell back, the floor began to pitch and roll, making it hard to stand steady, then it split in two, separating her from Miranda. A black putrid smoke spewed up from the chasm, followed by a bolt of white flame.

"General!" she cried, unable to see through the roaring wall of fire. All about her rocks and wood framing were falling and she could hear only their crashes, no one's voice. There was another rumble from the chasm of fire, and she felt herself falling toward it. "General!" she screamed, desperately thrusting her arms into the flames. Then she was jolted back by the firm grip of an arm about her waist.

Suddenly, she was lying in half recline across the red Moroccan seat of an open carriage. A white diaphanous gown clung to her body, her hair was dressed with blue flowers and long ribbons. The sky was cloudless, the sun beat heavily down, the air was sultry. Despite the high speed at which the driver paced his six Arabian horses, she began to perspire, her gown sticking to her thighs and stomach, each spot making her dress more transparent. "Driver," she called him, but he only whipped the steeds harder, his white shirt billowing in the wind, his thick black hair flying behind as they raced up and down the rounded hills on the road. Pandora's stomach jumped with each descent and every time she tried to rise and climb up to the driver's perch, she was thrown back onto the seat. Then, without warning, the coachman drew up the horses, who reared and pawed the earth. She saw his strong arms and hands control the reins with sheer power, then he rose and turned to her, a broad dazzling smile across his dark, sensuous face. It was Leander, reaching out to her. Her ardent body yearned for him.

The familiar sound of the library door broke into the dream. Pandora sat up and threw off her cover without hesitation. She darted for the stair. *It's the general, he's returned.* Her bare feet were light and fleet on the iron steps. She held her breath, so swept up was she in the miracle of his return.

"General, how did you get here? I just saw you in my dream. You were in prison. There was an earthquake—" she said to the tall figure facing the fireplace, her state of wakefulness still incomplete.

He turned, the candle he held illuminating his face softly.

"Leander!" she said. "It's only you, I thought—"

"I'm sorry you're disappointed."

"No, no, not at all. It was just that I was having the strangest dream—and then the door woke me and naturally, well, being only half awake, I thought it was him."

She realized she was not making much sense and that Leander was only half listening. Yet he was looking at her with such close scrutiny that she was suddenly aware that she was only clad in her thin nightdress. Instead of turning away she stayed silently fixed to his gaze. Leander moved nearer to her. He put out his hand and embraced her around the back of her head, ever so deliberately drawing them together. When their lips joined, her body succumbed completely to his support. Her head filled with his aroma and images of their two figures joined in the embrace. Deftly he lifted her with his good arm. She gently took hold of him around the neck, taking care of his wounded shoulder. Then he carried her up the stairs. He placed her on the bed, kissing her forehead, cheeks, and her neck. She kept her eyes closed, yet she had a picture of him bending over her. She reached for his buttons and began to undress him. He caught her hand and kissed the tips of her fingers, the softness of his lips evoking a low moan in her. She rose and knelt down by the bed, pulling off one boot, then the other, looking at his face all the while, their stares melting to one. He kissed the top of her head and her earlobes. Then he reached around her and drew her back onto the bed.

"I want you," he said.

"I want you, too," she said, allowing herself to fall back under his long, powerful body.

"I love you," he said.

"And I you," she answered.

"When I thought of dying," he turned on his side and brought her head to his chest, "my only torture was that I would never see you again, that you would never know how I yearned for you, that I would never hold you or kiss you."

"Leander." His lips came to hers, open, and he filled her mouth with his kisses, much deeper than before. She lost all sense of weight in her body, she felt like she was floating slowly, dreamily above the room, above any world she knew. She felt completely joined to him and secure in his dominance.

"I want you to be my wife, Pandora."

"Yes, oh yes..." She trembled.

"As soon as my wound has healed, I will go back to my regiment. But when I return you will be here waiting."

"Leander," she said, opening her eyes and looking at his love-drenched face. "Leander my love, I don't know what to say. I'm so terribly confused. I know that I love you, that I want to be your wife, but I am also a doctor. And whether or not it was wise for me to become one in the manner in which I did is water under the bridge. The fact remains I am a trained physician and I feel a solemn obligation to fulfill that oath."

"I don't understand what you are talking about."

"Right now I am only a doctor inside my masquerade, inside James Barry. James Barry cannot be your wife, I need to be your wife and a doctor."

"Right now that's impossible. There are no women doctors," Leander said.

"But there is. I am one. I just need to find a way to reveal it." She got up and went to the window. The night air cooled the perspiration that had moistened her body. "Leander, what if, tomorrow morning, I go first thing to the office of the London Times, whereupon I will request an interview with the editor. Upon compliance I will reveal to said person the entire story of my past and will then proclaim myself the world's first woman doctor." She sat on the sill, quite proud of how promising the plan sounded out loud, but after an awkwardly long silence and the deliberate way in which Leander rose and began buttoning his shirt, she realized things were not going to go smoothly.

"What, may I ask," Leander said, "do you suppose the reaction to your amazing revelation will be?"

She did not like his tone and she felt at once cold and uncomfortable with her near nakedness. "I would imagine it will cause quite a stir." She laughed, and reached for the dressing gown flung over her chair. "A lot of incredulity, shock, disbelief and certainly a decent amount of denunciation. But in the end, after the appropriate verifications have been secured, and the germane persons have given their testimony, the irrefutable facts of my accomplishment will be undeniable and the powers that be will have no recourse but to accept and acknowledge that there exists among them, measured by their own standards and certifications, a female doctor and surgeon."

"Brava! Brava!" Leander clapped his hand against his leg. "I did not know that we had in our midst the great diva of 'The Opera Bouffe.' But you must forgive me, dear lady, if I, a lowly soldier, venture a medical observation. I fear, Doctor Barry, that your hours in the rank bowels of the dissecting theater have had a deleterious effect on the function of your cerebrum. Although, if you'll pardon my saying, I never felt this was your most stable organ in the first place."

Pandora felt her cheeks burning as Leander's sharp words struck her.

"Do you really believe, Pandora, that all five feet and seven stone of you will single-handedly cause the existing order and mind set of the British educational and medical establishments to come completely about-face simply by the immense weight of your singular and suspect revelation?" He put up his hand as she tried to interject a defense. "Do you really believe that once you have told your tale, they will eagerly and fully accept you as one of them without question? Perhaps you expect them to proffer an apology for any inconvenience you might have endured. Yes, you do! I can see by the surprised look on your face. What an astoundingly naive child you are!"

Leander picked up his boots and strode in two broad steps to within inches of her. She stood defiantly but without a defense as he put his face close to hers. "Let me tell you their response; it will be swift, sure and overwhelming. After they have heaped cries of charlatan, impersonator, deviant and guisard on you, they will crown you with the grand title of impostor. After all that I imagine and, not surprisingly so, expect that they will remand you to irons with the charge of criminal misrepresentation.

"I am shocked that it never occurred to you what the real consequences of your 'divine revelation' would be."

Leander turned away, then swirled around again, rearmed. "No, that's a lie, I am not shocked at your behavior in the least. It is typical of your self-involved view of all that surrounds you, which brings me to another point. What of Lord Buchan, or have you forgotten my father's friend? The very person who, against his own good judgment and with considerable risk, participated in this harebrained web of intrigue. No, you did not think for one second what your grand pronouncement might mean to him. You were far too busy seeing yourself praised and glorified as the tiller of new ground, the launcher of ships, the savior of fools, the saint of the future! To consider even those who risked their reputations, their very security for you."

She hated him. He had struck a deep truth. She had not thought through anything but her own immediate goal and certainly she had not wondered about its effect on others. Moments ago they had loved each other so deeply she wanted to give herself completely. Now she hated him for his truth and surely he must hate her for her lack of it. But never, never, would she give him his due.

"Naturally, I knew you would take this pessimistic and pizzicato view of things." Her calm voice masked the taut hardness she felt in the pit of her stomach. "I see that you are still obsessed with the idea of finding fault with me and, once discovered, you can't resist the opportunity to diminish." She walked past him, no longer sure she could contain her hurt if she faced him. "Wouldn't it be far better, and far more helpful, if you tapped the wealth of your imagination, rather than cling to your self-righteousness, and help me come up with a counter move, a sound scenario from which I might achieve my most heartfelt endeavor, which is to bring honor to this house, not just to myself alone."

His fist slamming her dresser rattled the mirror hanging above it. She whirled at its force. She had never seen him in a man's rage.

"Pandora, you are a terrible bitch!" Leander said with such vengeance, his frame vibrated from the strength of it.

"This is old, old ground, and it is my fervent wish we do not travel it again, but you seem compelled not to leave it buried under new growth. Lying! Deception! Conniving! These are not the bones which support the body of honor, therefore they cannot exist among the noble! Get it straight, once and for all, there is no place on this globe as it is presently arranged, known or otherwise, where the disclosure of your ugly deception would be embraced, allowing your acceptance under the oath of Hypocrates, as one of its fellows. Therefore, my foolish friend, you are left with the ruins of what you have built. You must either return to your perverse charade, or discard it forever and put James Barry back in his grave where he can rest in the peace he deserves!" The deafening stillness that followed was almost worse than the horrible new truth

Leander had shouted at her. Her head got heavy; she wanted to fall onto her bed and escape into sleep to avoid further onslaught.

"Start a life that can stand the light of day." Leander persisted, so close to her face, she could feel that his body was as hot as his temper. "One which will have real honor!"

"I may be a bitch, Leander, but a doctor I am and a doctor I will remain."

CHAPTER THREE

Capetown, South Africa was not at all as she had imagined, during her long and, as before, unseaworthy journey from England. Time had not cured her of seasickness and, just like the short journey across the channel years ago, she had suffered that humiliating malady a good deal of this trip, so that even when they had stopped at St. Helena to unload cargo and provisions, she had not had the strength to walk with the other passengers to the boundary of the grounds where the great Napoleon was confined, in the hope of perhaps seeing him take the air. She had just remained in her deck chair, miserably contemplating the next leg of her endless voyage and imagining as one so often does when disposition overpowers, all of the worst possible scenarios that might arise upon her arrival at the Cape. So it was a great relief to her not only to touch solid ground but to find this young town in an energetic state of evolution, and that the climate and surroundings were pleasant and inviting.

A genial, free man by the name of Dantzen had approached even before she had left her cabin for disembarkation, announcing he was to serve her while she remained here. He immediately took charge of things, hoisting several of her bags and leading her to a waiting carriage. There she sat comfortably enjoying all the benefits of terra firma, while he saw to her papers and remaining luggage. By the time they had set out for her cottage quarters, the sun was low to the sea. It cast an amber gold light against the flat-topped rock, which rose up and dominated the view from the harbor to the town. She began to change the bleak picture she had drawn aboard ship of this far and strange land.

The streets were pleasantly wide, and the houses and shops that walled either side were bright with many windows fronting the avenues. Pandora imagined large, airy rooms behind these facades. Each corner seemed to steal one yet another view of Table Bay, which protected the land from the open sea.

She watched the back of her servant as he negotiated the streets and squares with smooth ease. His neck was thick, joining to his head in a seamless loop from one shoulder up and over his shortly cropped salt and pepper hair to the other side. His back was broad and powerful, well muscled without angles. He swayed in rhythm with the movements of the carriage, never looking behind, always attending their progress.

Though the streets were near empty, Dantzen kept a slow, steady pace, but Pandora suspected his control was such that at another time if speed were essential he could negotiate this same course at a far greater pace and still keep her flying about. So far this quietly poised fellow impressed her favorably, a good omen, she hoped.

When they stopped at last in front of the boarding house, number twelve Heerengracht, Dantzen quickly helped Pandora to her rooms, leaving her to open the wide French door, which led to a small but lovely garden in the back. Then he returned immediately to the carriage and her waiting luggage.

A good deal of Pandora's apprehension and just about all of her residual seasickness were now gladly in her past. She sat on a chair in front of her garden and let the gentle air carry away the long journey and its many disturbances.

"Excuse me, doctor, sir?" Dantzen startled her, but only in his quiet approach. His voice was as smooth and even as was his efficiency. "The widow Sandenberg, your proprietress, wishes to offer you some tea and sandwiches. If you would like, I can bring them to you here."

"That would be just fine, Dantzen, but I would like a word with you first." Dantzen stood unperturbed while Pandora gathered her thoughts. "Since we will be working quite closely together, there are a few things I wish to get straight right off. Being in the medical branch of the service, it is certain I will be summoned at many an odd hour. It should be clear that I am always to be awakened without hesitation. But since I am a person who values privacy to the extreme, I will require that my rooms never be entered until you have heard my specific command to do so. I hope this is understood completely and that it will be fulfilled to the letter."

"I understand, sir, and will see that there is no oversight."

"I am also uncompromising in the area of sanitation and cleanliness. No matter the hour upon which I return from my duties, nor the circumstance or weather condition, these rooms, my clothing, and especially my medical instruments must be meticulously clean. Is that understood?"

"Understood," Dantzen said, not a glimmer of perturbation in his voice.

"In the past people have told me that I possess quite a temper, that I am apt to lash out before listening. I hope you will learn not to take it too seriously and that you will be stalwart enough to speak to me if you feel that my treatment of you at any time is unjust or untoward. I do not wish to have resentments fester as they tend to blossom into terrible bitterness. An appropriate time to avoid this unpleasantness can always be found.

"Now," she said, extending her hand, "that is all I have to say. I am sure we will get on splendidly."

"Yes, sir. I think so," Dantzen said, smiling broadly for the first time. "I will see to your tea, sir."

***

The breeze came through the doors, blowing the curtains. Pandora awoke and looked over at her blue dress uniform hanging on her butler, then at her shiny black boots, which Dantzen had polished mirror-high and placed side by side next to her stool. The three-inch heels gave them a strange unbalanced look, but she had determined that being a five-foot civilian doctor was one thing, being such a diminutive officer was quite another, so while still in England she had the boots taken to a cobbler and the old heels replaced with these high ones; plus, she'd ordered extra kapok padding to enhance the width of her shoulders. She rose from her nap, slipped into her jacket, and watched herself button it in the tall glass set by the corner window of her room. The extremity of width in her shoulders did give her more bearing, but no tailor's trick was going to convince anyone that she was the conventional representation of the military doctor.

The whole effect from the shoulders to the boots was one of a strange, even freakish fellow, and, no doubt, questions would abound. Pandora understood she had to rely on her faith in her medical skills in order to quiet the concerns which were inevitable. She believed if she was given time she would ultimately gain acceptance and put to silence any gossip. It was always the beginning that was fraught with danger, because she was going to be judged by appearance without deed.

With this in mind she carefully placed her cocked hat on her head and tightened the belt of her sword. Then giving a last look in the mirror, she set out on her walk to the governor's home to present herself and report for duty.

***

The house of Governor Somerset was well lit when Pandora approached. Through the windows she saw a group of men sitting around a table, thoroughly engrossed in conversation. This pleasant picture, however, did little to alleviate her apprehension. "Staff Surgeon James Miranda Barry to see the governor and report for duty," she said, to the startlingly handsome blond soldier who responded to her knock. "Here are my papers." She handed up her papers and immediately caught the disdainful look in his eye as he canvassed her.

"Step inside, sir. I am Governor Somerset's aide de camp, Josias Cloete."

When Pandora entered the foyer and stood the same ground as the aide, she was completely unencumbered by intimidation. The mantle of doctor had secured itself so deeply inside her that this cursory moment of condemnation rendered by one who surely placed all his faith on his grand physique, only gave rise to her dander and she started looking for a way to fight.

He had a strong, square jaw divided in neat halves by a cleft on the chin. His skin was smooth and taut over his well-honed cheekbones, and his forehead was interrupted at the perfect place by a thick growth of shiny, blond hair, which covered his head in gentle waves. His eyes were an extraordinary blue, pale in shade, but piercing in their look. His shoulders were broad and well developed, his back was perfectly straight, and he held himself so well that there was not a crease or wrinkle in the fabric of his uniform as it met the edge of his tapered waist.

There was an awkward delay as Pandora realized Cloete was giving her the same scrutiny she was applying to him. His head cocked from side to side with a quizzical expression in his eyes just like a curious dog tries to confront the incomprehensible. He then walked slowly and deliberately around her, completing one circumference, then another before he let out an explosive guffaw. "Van der Weghe, Lambert, Morris come at once! Sheridan, you miserable clown! This time you've really topped the lot."

As Cloete's friends rushed into the vestibule, Pandora stood in bewilderment. "Look at this, will you!" Cloete said gaily, almost poking Pandora's eye out with his long reach. "*This* is our new chief medical officer, just arrived from England!"

Two of the men broke out into belly laughs and slapped each other heartily on the shoulders. But one did not join in the joke at all. He stood looking at her with an expression of deep sympathy. He was very thin for his height, and his skin was white and transparent looking. He did look very much like an adolescent schoolboy except for the thin beard and an expression of understanding that defied immaturity. Pandora assumed he was the same age as the others but not of healthy constitution.

"You are funnier than your uncle, Sheridan," Cloete said, to the serious fellow. "But how dumb do you think I am that I'd fall for some little miss dressed in a uniform? Surely, you could have found someone of grander stature to pull off this trick. My humiliation would have been far more effective with the governor than this thin masquerade."

Every one of the terrible thoughts Pandora had on the ship was suddenly coming true. Here she was in the real world of soldiers and already a mockery.

"Sheridan, I'm a bit surprised at your carelessness. Why, this young maid has no manly traits at all. Her face is totally smooth, her features delicate, and that padding in her shoulders could stuff a dozen pillows. And will you have a look at these heels? Quite a touch. Here, little lady, let's have a look at those heels."

Pandora slapped Cloete across the face, leaving a large red mark.

"Sir! I am Dr. James Miranda Barry, the new staff surgeon at this post. My credentials and a letter of introduction from Lord Buchan to Lord Somerset—I would be most grateful if you would give these to your superior so that I may be presented in the appropriate manner."

Everyone stood spellbound by Pandora's actions.

"Josias," Sheridan said, stepping between Cloete and Pandora. "You have presumed incorrectly. It seems this gentleman is precisely who he says he is, and you have blundered quite resoundingly. I have no prior knowledge of this fellow, as you assume, so I fear we owe him an apology."

Cloete's faced turned a crimson that blended with the sharpness of Pandora's slap. His upper lip moistened, and he could barely articulate his words. "Sir, please exc—Mr. Sheridan is a great prankster, I thought—this was—"

"I doubt you ever had a thought," Pandora snapped, forcing her papers into his hands. "I do not accept your apology. Announce me to Lord Somerset at once and have your second contact my servant this evening. I demand the proper satisfaction of your grievous insult to my person and the whole uniform of the British medical corps."

CHAPTER FOUR

The African night held a quiet Pandora never expected. It was as if the earth had completely shut down in wait for the morning sun to call it back to life, Pandora ran her hand over the wooden handle of her Wheelstock pistol. She pointed it into the dark and fired. Even though it was unloaded, the noise assaulted the peaceful repose of the night.

General Miranda had given her this pistol and had taught both her and Leander how to use it. No doubt Leander had become quite a perfect marksman by now. She remembered how awkward he had been at first and how upset he had gotten, his face colorless with envy when she had proved superior right off. Riding, however, had been his strong suit, though she was a perfectly fine horseman. The lamp flickered, casting a long shadow against the wall of her hand holding the gun. She kept it steady and watched the image and tried the trigger again.

"It's Dantzen, sir, may I come in?"

"Yes, certainly Dantzen, you may."

"Dr. Barry sir, excuse me, but may I say my piece?"

"Go on."

"I've had a word with Mr. Sheridan, and everything's arranged. He says it is quite irregular having a black man as your second, but—seeing as you don't know anybody as yet, and as I am a free man—he, Mr. Sheridan that is, says that's acceptable."

"Very well, Dantzen, and all the other details have been sorted out?"

"Yes, Dr. Barry. Dawn, twenty paces, single shot, no reload."

"Fine."

Pandora put her pistol in the green case and snapped it shut.

"Excuse me, sir. Mr. Sheridan, the others are willing to call the whole thing off. Mr. Cloete is most anxious to make things right. He asked me again to extend his apology to you."

Pandora was unmoved by Cloete's repeated efforts to stave off the inevitable. She rose and went to her desk.

"You'll excuse me, sir, but if you ask me, the whole thing seems a bit foolish," Dantzen said.

"I didn't ask you, did I?" Pandora held up the black tin box she had carried from France. "If I am killed, you'll find a letter in this box which will contain some specific details for the disbursement of my possessions and personal wishes. Please see that it and my other belongings here are returned to London as quickly as possible and that no one but yourself handles things."

"As you say, sir. You will be leaving in about a half hour. Would you like some food before the carriage is brought round?"

"No, let's go now. I'd like to walk in the field awhile before the others arrive." Pandora put her gloves on, and Dantzen secured her dress spurs. She wore her entire dress uniform so that in the event she was killed, she would be appropriately attired.

As the carriage left the front of her boarding house, then departed the confines of the city streets and headed to the open countryside, Pandora watched the waning night sky, the stars disappearing until it seemed the heavens had very few. A pale hint of rose just washed the eastern horizon, and the moon looked more and more like a dark thumb smudge on a canvas than the great night illumination it was. Somehow none of these things affected her differently than they would on any usual morning. She had no sense of strangeness toward the normal evolutions of night to day despite the fact that this day could well be her last, that this hour could well be her last. Somehow she felt right that, whatever the outcome, she knew it was destiny that held her in the wave of its control. God's resolve seemed at hand, and she was supplicantly receptive to His sovereignty.

Early on she had vowed she would only attempt to wound Mr. Cloete. She would aim for the thigh and strike flesh, avoiding shattering a bone. Of course, she hoped it would be her bullet which would hit first, but she allowed her first instinct for revenge in the extreme to cool, and this second thought seemed correct, even if she ran a greater risk of her own death.

"We're here, Dr. Barry." Dantzen stopped the carriage on top of a gentle, grassy hillside, which glided down in compliant rolls to the edge of a large lake. At the far end antelope were drinking and, save for the occasional chirp of a restless bird, all was still. Pandora walked a short way down the incline, breathing in the clear air and opening and closing her right hand. Then the sound of another carriage filled the air. She saw Dantzen looking down at her, only a silhouette at the top of the hill. Then an open carriage appeared just behind him. There were two horses pulling it and four men aboard.

Mr. Cloete always makes a point to impress, she thought. When she reached the top, Cloete was at the lip of the carriage, draped in a long black cape. His head was covered in a wide-brimmed hat, also black. When he removed both hat and cape, his erect posture and serious expression made him seem even more handsome than before.

"Dr. Barry?" Mr. Sheridan said, discreetly, over Pandora's shoulder. "We can still call this off and no one be embarrassed. After all, sir, I have the somewhat dubious distinction of being the colony's resident jokester, and Mr. Cloete knows it only too well. His remarks were not at all intended with malice, they were of the most unprejudiced innocence."

"I am prepared. I assume your man is as well."

Dantzen stood by Pandora with the pistol box as Mr. Van der Weghe explained the procedure. Cloete's eyes expressed no fear but showed deep concern. Clearly he felt at the advantage.

"Ready?" Morris called. Dantzen handed Pandora her gun. She held it up at her shoulder and turned her back to Cloete. "One, two." Pandora began her pace with each command, her surety of purpose gaining as the distance between her and Cloete grew. "Eighteen, nineteen, twenty, turn! Fire!"

Her arms drew straight as she turned to face him. His height gave her a perfect bead. She aimed precisely at the chest, but instantly lowered to the right thigh and fired. She heard his report and felt at once something pass over her head. But at that second she saw him bend down onto one knee, then go to a sit on the ground. Her bullet had struck.

"My bag in the carriage," Pandora ordered Dantzen, as she rushed to Cloete, her heart beating hard. She pushed aside Morris and Sheridan and fell to her knees. Dantzen put the bag down beside her. Blood was spreading in a long oval stain on Cloete's white breeches. She cut the pant. Thank God, she thought, the bullet had perfectly struck, missing the bone entirely. "You shot over my head," she said, cleaning and stuffing the wound as best she could.

"I had hoped you'd do the same," Cloete said.

"Well, I didn't, did I? You damned fool." She stretched his leg out and wrapped the dressing. "Take him to my quarters. I'll properly dress the injury there."

"Yes, Dr. Barry," Morris, Sheridan, and Van der Weghe said in unison.

CHAPTER FIVE

"You really are a stubborn bastard, James," Captain Cloete said, his hands crossed over his broad chest. "I don't like this warden—Dennysen—any more than you do, but to drag him here from his house on a Sunday, over the matter of this lunatic, seems to me to carry the game a bit too far."

"No one insisted you come, Josias. I am perfectly capable of handling the matter on my own," Pandora said.

The Tronk Prison office where they sat, though large and airy, was nonetheless drab and uninviting. It was rendered thus by the sparseness of its furnishing and lack of color on its walls. There were the two chairs which they now occupied, a stark wooden file cabinet, and the warden's fastidiously neat desktop with his straight-backed chair.

"Indeed you are quite capable of handling things. When it comes to making influential enemies, my friend, no one is your equal."

"I am merely doing my job." Pandora smiled wryly at her former dueling partner's remark.

"Excuse my tardiness, gentlemen." Daniel Dennysen, the Lord Fiscal of Cape Town, shut the door. "Surely I do not understand the need for both you lads to interrupt the pleasures of a glorious Sunday with such a matter as we have here."

Pandora watched as he took some papers from a desk drawer and tapped them even on the desk.

"These documents simply require your signature, for which I would gladly have sent my aide rather than cause inconvenience." Dennysen was not much taller than Pandora and razor-thin. He was all neatness and order from his perfectly slicked-back brown hair, of which he had a considerable amount for a man of his fifties, to his clipped speech and perfectly fitted suit.

Pandora didn't move to take the papers and the warden spoke again.

"From my personal observation of Mr. Smith, the prisoner, I can assure you he is an extremely dangerous madman, not safe to himself or anyone else here at Tronk Prison." Dennysen smoothed the papers on his desk and dipped his quill pen into the well. "Inspector, you can see these commitment papers are all in order and require only our two signatures." He signed his name and pushed both pen and paper toward Pandora. "If you'll place your signature below mine, we can terminate this matter post haste and return to our homes to enjoy the remainder of the Lord's day."

"I admire your thoughtfulness and your dedication, Mr. Dennysen," Pandora said, making no gesture to take the quill. "Heaven only knows where we would be if all public servants rose to their responsibility with as much sincere fervor as yourself. It is a doctor's lot to expect such inopportune interruptions, as illness and pain take no respite. But your sacrifice of a day with loved ones for this prisoner's well being is far more virtuous. Yet, since we have all found our way here, whatever the justification, we might as well have a look around since I have not as yet inspected this part of my jurisdiction. While I am looking at this, Mr. Smith, I may as well examine the others, perhaps perform some small service to another poor soul whose difficulties, despite your diligence, may have gone unnoticed. What better day to do the Lord's work than on the Sabbath?"

Pandora rose, ignoring Dennysen's tightening jaw.

"This is quite unnecessary, gentlemen," Dennysen said. "You have my word that everything under this roof is in strict conformity to His Majesty's law. And within those regulations established by his excellency, Lord Somerset, as well."

"While I am sure everything is just as you say it is," Cloete said, "Dr. Barry relies on his own personal observation in these matters, because as a medical man he might make some observations that those with an untrained eye – despite noble intentions – might overlook or misinterpret."

"If you will be so kind and lead the way, I would like to proceed before we lose the daylight," Pandora said, bag in hand.

When they passed through the first wood door and approached the guard gate separating the office complex from the prison itself, Pandora thought of Haly, Mathilde and all the souls that had drawn her to the French prisons every day. When the big iron gate yawned and groaned, allowing them into the murky corridor, flanked by heavy cell doors forbiddingly closed and bolted, she automatically felt great sympathy and support for those incarcerated, even though she knew it was probably naive thinking.

As they neared the cell in question horrible howls could be heard from within. A bruin-like Hottentot guard who stood outside banged the butt of his stick three times against the cell door and threw back the observation slot. "Shut your yap, you batty bastard. There're important gentlemen here to see you. Behave yourself or I'll come in there and teach you some fine manners."

The prisoner threw something against the door with such force it shocked its bolts and locks, startling Dennysen, who stepped three paces back, prompting a grin from the guard. "This is our prized loony. Have a look for yourself," the guard said.

Pandora looked inside but the light was so scant and the man's movements so agitated she could make out few features other than his nakedness and his knotty-muscled frame. "You see, gov," said the guard, "his ding-dong chimes is ringin' off-key."

Mr. Smith screamed.

Pandora caught the filthy smell from inside the cell. She looked hard through the barred window.

"Open the door," she said.

"Just give me a minute, gov, and I'll quiet him down for you so you can have a nice easy visit."

"You'll do nothing of the kind. Just open the door. I'm going in alone."

"I'll not take responsibility for juvenile bravado," Dennysen said, from behind her.

"This isn't wise, James," Cloete said.

"I do believe I ordered that door opened. I am waiting."

The guard slipped the bolt and moved the chain, allowing the door to open a crack. Pandora silently stepped into the dark cell, Cloete right behind her. They stopped just inside, close to the wall. Opposite them, frozen still, was Mr. Smith. He was stark naked, manacled at his ankles and wrists. He was covered with sweat and ulcerated sores. Pandora also saw that one leg was horribly swollen and bore a dark, nearly black mark on the upper thigh. His mouth was contorted by swelling and encrusted with dried blood. His eyes were wild and tormented, seeming to shriek out in their gaze.

Suddenly he threw his head back and howled long and loud, like some deeply forlorn animal. Cloete attempted to put himself between Smith and Pandora.

"Stay back," she said, handing him her bag. "This is fear you're witnessing, not viciousness." Then Pandora threw her head back and identically imitated the seaman's howl. Mr. Smith grabbed the slop pail and heaved it at Pandora and Cloete, drenching them with the filth inside.

Without pause and with the same two-handed motion, Pandora threw it back, letting it hit the wall behind him. Smith crouched down, grabbed some straw, and screaming all the while, threw it at his intruders and all about the cell. Pandora followed suit. Then the two of them, Pandora taking his lead, but all the while drawing closer to him, began running back and forth from one side of the small cell to the other, hitting the walls with their shoulders, their howls finally reaching one unified crescendo. When Pandora was quite close, the seaman stopped abruptly and started panting. Pandora panted with him.

"Flablah—flamight."

Pandora listened and mimicked his words, trying to make some sense for him as well as herself.

"Flablah—flamight," he repeated.

Pandora lowered the intensity. "You're a seaman, Mr. Smith, you're a seaman." Smith started to let his body slump, his legs bending, the chained hands dropping. "You're a seaman," Pandora repeated. "Think of the open sea." Pandora was now within inches of Mr. Smith, his body slackened, he dropped submissively to his knees. Pandora followed him again and placed her hand on his soaked, scarred shoulder. He flinched abruptly at her touch, but immediately relaxed.

"I just want to die," he moaned. "Please, help me die."

She removed her jacket, rolled it to a pillow and guided Smith's head to the ground. "My bag." Cloete was already there and placed it beside her. She removed her scalpel.

"Why do they treat me this way? Why do they beat me so? I'm only a drunken fool."

"Burns," she cursed. Pandora opened several festering blisters on the man's back and expressed fluid.

The guard noisily dropped a pail of water near her. She washed Mr. Smith's oozing sores. "Mr. Dennysen," she called, "come in here. It's perfectly safe. I want you to observe something."

Dennysen timidly appeared, keeping himself securely behind the guard. Pandora rose and took the guard's large hand and placed her own inside his palm.

"Mr. Dennysen, observe these two hands. Our friend here obviously has the larger and no doubt the stronger. No doubt, Mr. Dennysen, our brave guard does not hesitate to use this large and powerful hand in the discharge of his manly duties." She patted the guard's arm. "Now gentlemen, observe my rather small and weak hand." She made some graceful movements with her hand, pushing the air gently away. "Not very large, not very strong. However, the difference between my hand and the appendage of our guard is that mine is attached to a brain." With a lightning swift motion, Pandora whipped her scalpel to the neck of the stunned and perplexed guard.

"My God!" Dennysen gasped.

"Do you know sir, at which part of your anatomy I have placed my knife?"

"My throat, doctor. D-don't cut my throat," stammered the guard.

"To be exact, this instrument of justice is poised just above your carotid artery, which connects your poor excuse for a heart to that rudiment you call a brain."

"Captain Cloete, I demand you put a stop to this shameful display at once!" shrieked Dennysen.

"By exerting the slightest pressure, I can quickly and painlessly end your life." Pandora flicked her wrist. A gasp came from Mr. Smith, who lay calm on her jacket.

"Ach!" the guard grabbed his throat with a trembling hand and looked at the trickle of blood coming from where Pandora had nicked him.

"You see gentlemen, the ultimate power in this room rests in these small quick hands. Fascinating, is it not? Now, Mr. Dennysen—?" She met him with a cold, hard stare. "Captain Cloete and I will inspect each and every one of these holes you call cells, and if this man is touched again, I will dissect the one who is responsible."

CHAPTER SIX

"Dancin's the way to get yourself a woman, doctor," Van Helfin said, his thickset body swaying just short of uncontrollability. His rough and ready Dutch complexion was rosier than the norm, thanks to his all too frequent trips to the punch bowl. Pandora, in her blue dress uniform, listened tolerantly, two cups hooked through her fingers. "And there you are, graced on either side with not one, but two handsome fillies. And them being the governor's daughters at that. My, my." The drunken fellow cast a rude glance across the dance floor where Pandora had just left Lord Somerset and his two daughters. She had just filled her cups with the vermilion colored punch and was attempting escape. "Aren't you the lucky rogue?" Van Helfin winked.

"Indeed so. He's a popular fellow," said Van Helfin's scarecrowish partner, Landdrost Van der Groot, whose wheat colored hair was so closely cropped one could see his scalp through it. "But if it were me, I'd not be here jabbering or standing away far off neither. No, son, you won't find your way into the promised land that way," he said, clasping Pandora's shoulder with a viselike grip. The band resumed its strains with a punctual minuet. The women's gowns rustled and stirred up the breeze as they moved in and out with their partners.

"No, lad," said Van Helfin, his liquor-soaked breath preceding his words. "When you move a woman round and round, that's what makes them hot."

"Like I said," overlapped Van der Groot, "if t'were me, I'd never be still a moment. I'd exchange one for the other at each turn of the band all night through. By Jesus, who the hell knows?" Van der Groot puckered his mouth close to Pandora's ear. "Maybe you could get lucky with both," he said, spraying a ribald laugh in her face, while Van Helfin drained another cup.

"I find," Pandora said, "your concern for my mating quite charming. But may I assure you, gentlemen, that there are other things to do in life than to spend all your time and energy hoping to be stuck together like dogs on a June night. I must inform you that the finely rendered music and pleasant conversation of two jeunes demoiselles, such as the daughters' Somerset, is satisfaction enough."

"Well, he thinks himself a popular fellow, doesn't he?" Van Helfin turned back for another ladle of punch as Van der Groot watched Pandora weave in and out among the dancers, wending her way toward Lord Somerset, his two daughters and Captain Cloete. "But there are some nasty stories going round about him and Captain Cloete," Van Helfin said. "Quite a team they've been since that duel. That little fellow certainly knows how to make friends."

"And enemies," Van der Groot interjected. "But as long as he's the governor's physician..."

"Yes, well, he's in love with him, too, ever since he fixed up Miss Georgiana when she come down with the rot koorts." Van Helfin watched the bustle that always occurred whenever Pandora passed any of the gatherings of people.

"How's the sea-bathing affecting your rashes?" she said, stopping to acknowledge the wife of the burgher, who had been plagued with skin rashes.

"Quite satisfactory, Dr. Barry, and the diet seems to ease them as well."

"He's a remarkable chap indeed." Pandora heard a woman in the group acknowledge as she moved away from them.

"Ah, Dr. Barry, I was just talking about you and the recovery you brought about with my youngest daughter. Why, she has slept these past three nights without being awakened by that horrible cough."

"Excellent, Mrs. Smeadly," Pandora said. "Discontinue the poultice in the morning and render one application at bedtime. I am glad the child is better, but don't allow her too much activity for several days hence."

"Oh, doctor, we've never seen one the likes of you here. You're a miracle man, you are."

"I'm afraid miracles are not in my line, but thanks for the compliment nonetheless."

"Dr. Barry, these are some dear friends of mine whom I want you to meet. They've already heard many wonderful things about you.."

***

"Well, one day," Van Helfin stood at the edge of the dance floor, talking half to himself. "He won't have so many archangels looking out for him. Then he'd better watch out."

"Strange lot, the British," Van der Groot joined in.

***

"If you gain one drop more in popularity James, I'm afraid there'll be a populist movement to make you governor," said Lord Somerset, as Pandora finally reached her host and handed the two punch glasses to the ladies.

"You have no need to fear that, your excellency. My detractors may be fewer in number than my supporters, but their passion and their power, at least, make for a balance."

"Dr. Barry, it is always a mistake to give malicious gossip a passing thought," Georgiana Somerset said. She was the elder girl, quite tall, with thick shiny auburn hair, a straight narrow nose, oval cat eyes of a yellowish green and a long willowy neck.

The band struck a lively tune. Captain Cloete gave his arm to Charlotte Augusta, Lord Somerset's younger daughter, a softer beauty than her sister, fair-haired and peach-skinned, her blue eyes always twinkling as if she were ready to laugh at any moment. Pandora watched as Cloete took her waist and drew her round. She relented with such ease and took up his lead in so smooth a way it seemed the two had done nothing other than practice their dancing day in and day out.

Whenever she tilted her head back Josias would lean toward her and, whatever he might be saying, Pandora saw that Charlotte always turned a bit flushed around her ears and neck and let her laughing eyes look away. Pandora could not take her eyes away from them and despite herself she was jealous. It was utterly absurd for her to feel Josias was hers. But she did and no matter how severely she admonished herself about the insanity of these ideas, nothing contained the beast.

The band broke into a spirited clog dance. Pandora captained the line of men on one side while Georgiana served as counterpart with the women. Pandora began with strong heel-toe movements, letting her body lean into each tap and stomp for greater accent. Georgiana followed from the other line, forcing the band to play louder. Pandora's jealousy spurred her on. As the music stepped up she increased her speed and the band followed.

The other dancers, unable to keep up, moved to the sidelines and became spectators. Soon Pandora was leading Georgiana in one large skipping circle. They created a stage in the middle of the dance floor. When they reached the center of it Pandora put both hands on Georgiana's waist and the bright tempo of the song leapt to a wilder, more furious pace. They began to spin and stomp, and, sidestepping at all the right spots, Pandora could see only the blur of the crowd around them as they kept up their challenge with the music. Then, with an abrupt crescendo, the band punched a stop. Pandora pulled Georgiana in about the waist and they gracefully slowed to a smooth halt. The crowd burst into cheers and applause. Pandora swung Georgiana out into a curtsy and bowed herself. A waltz began.

"May I have this waltz?" a tall, youthful officer said to Georgiana.

"By all means," Pandora said, relinquishing Georgiana to the handsome fellow. "The closer I get to the feet of my partner, the more dangerous I become." She said, looking around until she saw Captain Cloete swirling smoothly with Charlotte in perfect pace.

CHAPTER SEVEN

The driving rain beat down on the drum-taut roof of the carriage. The cobble stones submitted under its speeding wheels. Pandora held tight the hand grip above her head, as Dantzen encouraged his pair up the long driveway. She glanced out and saw light spilling from the doorway of the stately manor, framing the solitary figure of its squire, Thomas Munnik. "Thanks to Heaven, you are here!" he said, ignoring the drench streaming down his anxious face and soaking his jet black hair. Pandora leapt from her carriage and rushed up the three short steps for the cover of the Georgian veranda, which swept across the face of the residence. "This way, please hurry, Doctor. I don't know how much longer she can hold out. I don't care about the child," he said, leading her inside. "Please just save my wife." Pandora could see that his jovial face was unaccustomed to the wear and fatigue it now bore so uneasily.

"I'll do everything I can," she said, removing her black cape to the waiting servant. As they passed from the foyer to the stair, Pandora did not fail to notice the open grandeur of the living room, which, despite Mrs. Munnik's grave situation, kept its cheery and expectant appearance, with fresh cut flowers and her half finished needlework stretched in its frame across from Mr. Munnik's reading chair.

"The nurse, Mrs. McNamara, has been with her night and day since the confinement began five days ago," explained Munnik, as they reached the second floor landing. "But now that the others have given her up, she can only soothe her. Since any positive signs have all but halted in the last day, you are our final hope, sir." He rushed past Pandora, into the softly lit bedchamber. She watched him take his wife's pale hand into his and kiss her fingers imploringly.

"I am Nurse McNamara, Dr. Barry," said the leathery matron, abandoning her chair at the foot of Mrs. Munnik's bed and extending a stiff hand. "This unfortunate situation must soon come to an end. All the others have told him so. I don't know why Mr. Munnik bothered to bring you out. The little creature inside has nowhere near enough room to make his escape. There is nothing that can be done."

"Mr. Munnik," Pandora said, approaching the bed, "you can serve best if you'll leave us now to do our task." The merchant rose from his knee at Pandora's words. The drops of rain transported by his coat, leaving a ring on the rich Persian carpet, where he had knelt.

"Whatever is best," he said, anguish blurring his dark eyes.

"A mild libation will do you some good," Pandora said.

"Thomas, please try not to worry so." Gwendolyn Munnik put out her feeble hand and touched her husband's trouser. Despite her wan face and decidedly weakened state, Pandora saw she was a determined woman and thus encouraged she was anxious for Mr. Munnik to leave the two of them alone.

"Dr. Barry is here now, dear husband. You can be easy, for he is known to work miracles."

"I only care about you, my dearest—my beloved," Thomas said.

"Mr. Munnik, please, you must leave now," Pandora said.

He leaned over and stroked his wife's cheek with his lips. "God bless, my darling," he whispered, and began to back out of the room, but emotion overtook him and he started back to his wife's bed.

"Nurse!" Pandora said.

"Come along, Mr. Munnik, some prayers for the Lord's strength are what you need," the nurse said. "This carrying on only makes it worse." She wrapped his stooped frame with her big arm and led him away. Pandora stood aside contemplatively assessing her patient.

"Please, Thomas, go along. You men are of no use at all in these times. Isn't that the truth, Doctor?" She smiled faintly.

"Quite true, Madame," Pandora said, but her thoughts were

piecing together another puzzle, as she took note of Gwendolyn Munnik's condition. Though her physical constitution was precariously weakened from days of fruitless labor, Pandora marveled at the spiritual courage, a kind of "mother's morale" which seemed to lift her away from the parapet of defeat.

She pulled back the heap of covers and lifted the young woman's nightdress, going about her examination full of thought and tender hands. "You can speak frankly with me, Doctor," Mrs. Munnik said, in a fragile but steady way. "I know they've given up all hope for us."

Pandora placed her hand on the woman's troubled womb. She felt the hardness and her thoughts began to congeal. "I insisted they call you," Mrs. Munnik continued, despite Pandora's uncomfortable prods. "I have heard so much about you and so many have such faith in you. Don't ask me why, but I just know you can save us."

Pandora sat down on the bed. "Tell me," Gwendolyn asked as Pandora covered the woman's hand with hers, "would it have been better to send for a minister than a doctor?" Before Pandora could respond, Mrs. McNamara returned.

"I do apologize for sending you back and forth, nurse, but I need something of a special, medical nature for Madame."

"Of course, Doctor."

"Would you bring us a glass of the very finest sherry that Mr. Munnik might have?"

"Yes, doctor, right away," she said, a bit on the perturbed side. "I'll bring it right along."

"Mrs. Munnik," said Pandora.

"Gwendolyn, please call me by my Christian name."

"Very well, Gwendolyn. You and I must now speak plainly, for time is exceedingly precious." Pandora felt just a start of fright pass through Mrs. Munnik's hand. "The others are quite right. This child will not arrive in the world in the usual way. But there is a hope, if we pursue another course of action."

"I don't understand." Gwendolyn said.

"We must remove the child surgically from the womb," Pandora said, looking steadily at her patient, whose faded eyes then rose to a glow. Encouraged, Pandora interpreted this as a stoic acceptance, which this woman seemed to possess or perhaps possessed her.

"Do what you must, Doctor. My child and I are in your hands."

Pandora at once began her preparation, rearranging candles, lamps and furniture, just as the nurse again returned with Mrs. Munnik's sherry. "Ah, your tonic has arrived. Now Mrs. McNamara, have the servants bring a sturdy table and as much light as can be provided."

"What are you going to do, doctor?" the bewildered nurse asked.

"Operate!" snapped Pandora.

"I've never heard of such a thing!" McNamara said.

"Just do as you are told, and be quick about it."

McNamara stormed to the door, but Pandora was unaffected. Her mind was full of preparation and anticipation. "You must understand, Gwendolyn," she said, handing her the sherry, "this will cause you considerable pain, but I am skillful and quick, and if you think of the great reward which will be closed in your embrace at the end, all will pass easier."

"My God!" shouted Munnik, Nurse McNamara at his heels. "You'll kill her! What is this madness you're proposing? You're a madman!" He went to his wife and stood between her and Pandora. "You cannot cut her open! Why, it's unholy! I thought I'd sent for a doctor, not a butcher!" Pandora's ire flashed both at Mr. Munnik and the insubordinate nurse who stood at his side.

"Sir, you summoned me after all others have failed to save your wife and unborn child. That is exactly what I intend to do, with Mrs. Munnik's full and lucid understanding. Now I will no longer tolerate another such interruption, or you will have to accept my withdrawal from this case and take on your own shoulders whatever the consequences."

"Thomas, come," Gwendolyn said. "Leave me alone with Dr. Barry. We must allow him to proceed."

"But you—?" Munnik asked, unable to say the rest.

"I am ready," she said. "Now let the job be done."

Obediently, he retired, allowing the servants to bring Pandora a table and arrange the lamps and candle stands around it. Nurse McNamara joined in, a prejudiced but competent assistant. "You know, Gwendolyn," she said, "the last time I did this I pulled a carved doll out of a pillowcase."

When Mrs. Munnik was laid on the table, Pandora handed her the glass of sherry. Then she took up her scalpel and made the first incision. She worked with lightning speed, following exactly the steps she had practiced in the "Dead House" at Edinburgh. "Hold her steady," she ordered the nurse and servants. "We're almost there, Gwendolyn." Mrs. Munnik bore her pain majestically, her total concentration like Pandora's, on the success of delivery.

"Here we are!" Pandora suddenly exclaimed, lifting high a rather worn and withered newborn. There was a wail and a whimper at the infant's first breath. "You have born a man child," Pandora said, handing the infant to Nurse McNamara. Then, with deft surety, Pandora began to stitch the incision. The long reserved tears flowed quietly but freely from Gwendolyn Munnik's eyes. "I am not quite finished with you, Madame," Pandora said, drawing back her own emotion.

"Go right ahead, Dr. Barry," the patient said above the infant's free and welcome wails. "You have brought me, my son, James Barry Munnik. He will keep my mind free of pain or impatience."

***

"Dr. Barry, how can I ever show my gratitude? What can I do to repay you? Anything I have is yours."

Pandora laughed at Mr. Munnik's confused behavior. His round figure darted from one side of the room to the other, as if he were looking for some great treasure to take up and present to her with royal gesture. "Mr. Munnik, I have been repaid many fold by the fact that we were able to save your wife and the child. And she has given the boy my name, a gift of more staying power and significance than any monies or materials you might give me. But I do think it is advisable for me to remain here the night and as I am quite exhausted, I would be most grateful for a soft bed and some warm water to wash myself."

"I had anticipated your wish, Dr. Barry. A warm tub is just now being drawn, and I think the room will be of satisfaction. I thought Cook could bring you a small supper if you wish. You must be ravenous." Mr. Munnik led Pandora down a pastel-painted corridor lined with small drawings and lighted by several sconces. "Food is not necessary, sir, but would you let Mr. Dantzen know I am retiring and that he may return home."

"Yes, indeed," Munnik said, opening the door to a cozy room stuffed with figurines, framed floral prints, a charming canopy bed, several chairs with brocade seats, and a handsome maple dresser. "Inside there," Mr. Munnik pointed to two mirrored doors, "you will find your tub. I'll see to Mr. Dantzen now. Good night."

"Good night, Mr. Munnik."

Pandora finished her tub and slipped on her cotton shirt, leaving it open as it was no longer raining and the air was soothing. She picked up a book of poems from one of the little clusters of books arranged on the night table and lay down on the top of the bed. She began to read, but quickly everything faded as her body sank into the bed's softness. The quiet room and the pleasant light lulled her to a gentle sleep. She did not hear the first or second knock on the door, and before "wait" could come from her lips or she was able to cover herself, she saw Nurse McNamara standing in the doorway.

"Oh, my God in heaven! You're a woman!" she said, in horror.

Pandora sprang from the bed and turned her back to the flabbergasted nurse, buttoning her shirt and grabbing her trousers. "What is it? Is Mrs. Munnik in need of me," she said, over her shoulder. "What is it? Why have you simply barged in here without knocking, you damned fool?"

"But, Doct–, ah, um, I did, I had no idea you were a worn–, I mean, I came to say Captain Cloete is here to see you.

"Indeed," Pandora said, buttoning her pants. "You listen to me. I don't know what you think you saw when you barged in here. But if there's any foolishness about it, I'll cut your ears clean off."

"Yes, Doctor." McNamara said, scurrying from the room.

CHAPTER EIGHT

The morning was crisp, the sky a deep blue at the horizon, so that the hills and slopes were sharply defined at their point of meeting. Pandora filled her lungs with fresh air and patted her black poodle, Psyche, on the top of the head. Psyche licked her hand and darted out onto the sidewalk, turning north in the exact direction of Saunders's Confectioner. Every morning after Pandora returned from rounds, the two had this ritual. Pandora would take the dog with her and they would walk to the confectioner's where she would buy two sweet buns, and then they would return home. But ever since the miraculous events at the Munniks' a year ago, Pandora's usually quiet and private walk had become a symphony of greetings, stares, and awed confrontations. From Dutch to Hottentot, she'd be stopped many times to respond to a question or receive a salutation or just be stared at. So celebrated was she that the newspapers carried stories of her various exploits. Her public seemed insatiable always clamoring for more. The journals had taken to exaggerating her practices quite enthusiastically, so that when she had gone to St. Helena to treat one of Emperor Napoleon's staff members for an eruption of boils (blood fever), it was naturally reported that she had been there to treat Bonaparte himself and that wondrous secrets had been exchanged.

Later, when she had been summoned to help treat an outbreak of cholera in Mauritius, her dispatches from there were posted and read by all with the fervor of a populace receiving word from their general waging war at the front. When she vehemently reformed the treatment of the lepers at Hemel-ard by demanding proper diet and constant cleaning and treatment of the poor creatures' sores, there circulated stories among the native population that her magic was so strong she could actually cure the malignant malady. This widespread acclaim translated into power and she used it like a sword.

She cut a wild figure with her cockaded hats, her overly broad shoulders and lifted boots, as she walked regularly about town, Psyche at her heel. Oftentimes Dantzen would follow holding an umbrella above her head to protect her from the sun. The Hottentots referred to her as the Kapok Doctor, due to her exceptional shoulder padding, but their attitude was far from irreverent.

Whenever and wherever Pandora felt the established order of the colony was insalubrious to the public weal, she attacked with vigor. She had cracked down hard on the indiscriminate sale of patent medicines and attacked the system of nepotism among the apothecaries, which had until then been the practice by which one attained a license.

In this way the young officer had acquired not only admirers and devotees but sincere and powerful enemies. Though these were few in number, they were dedicated to her downfall and they had coalesced into an ad hoc cabal with the vindictive Dennysen at the head. Pandora was far from unaware of this situation; her friends constantly warned her, pointing out that her enemies were not to be underestimated. But the combination of hotheaded youth, accomplishment, and acclaim made her feel impregnable. She felt herself a match for death itself and saw no need whatever to fear a few small-minded, conniving men.

Just as Psyche reached the door of the house, the little bag of buns clenched in his teeth, Josias Cloete's carriage drew up in front. The dog, recognizing his friend, began jumping and prancing in little circles with enthusiasm.

"Is there anything in that bag for me," Cloete said, opening the door of the carriage. Psyche leapt inside and onto his lap, bag of buns and all. Pandora laughed as the two exited the carriage, Cloete now carrying the bag of buns under the watchful eyes of Psyche. "Good morning, James, I trust our chief medical officer approves of this weather."

"Just as I prescribed," Pandora said. "And you seem in fine fettle this morning."

"Tip top," Cloete said.

"Well then, what is it that brings you by so early?"

"I came to tell you about a meeting with Governor Somerset this afternoon. There seems to be quite a stir over some of your latest proposals, vis-a-vis the Leper colony. There are some who don't quite appreciate your zeal—Mr. Dennysen and Sir Richard Plaskett in particular. And while the governor has taken your part, he will need you to defend your position in person."

"You worry far too much, Josias. It's not good for your health. Come in and have tea." Pandora followed Psyche into her sitting room. Dantzen was just arranging the tea and Psyche, having reached his limit of patience, began yelping at Dantzen to place a bun on his dish.

"Yes, yes, Psyche. I know what 'tis you want, but the doctor and Captain Cloete have got to have the tea hot, so it will be a minute more."

Psyche appeared to understand precisely what Dantzen had said, because he sat right down and followed the servant's every move in total silence.

"Oh," Cloete said. "I almost forgot entirely, I've brought you a letter from London."

Pandora blushed when she saw the hand was Leander's. She had not heard from him and had only followed his whereabouts from Sarah, who gave news of his well-being in her letters. In her expectancy, she stood up, then sat down again quickly.

"Would you rather I leave?" Cloete said.

"Oh no, Josias." She let out one of those uncontrollably foolish giggles, but covered it with a cough just as fast. "Please, stay. I want to hear more about this meeting. I'll just take a moment." She tore open the letter, a picture of Leander growing in her mind.

My dear Pandora,

It is with laborious effort and a grief-stricken heart that I write to you the blackest of news. My father, your beloved general, has passed from his

Spanish prison to his final and deserved reward. Death has become his liberator.

Pandora gasped and quickly stuffed the letter in her pocket.

"Is it bad news?" Cloete asked, but Pandora had already moved toward the terrace. Her head had suddenly become a storm of thoughts and images. The past began to tumble in uncontrollably, and a terrible lump began to build in her chest.

"Can I do anything," Pandora heard Josias ask. "No, thank you, but I would like to be left alone, if you don't mind." She only heard the door close.

As I put these words to paper, I wish I could have softened their effect with my presence. But our great distance both physically and spiritually has obliterated such a possibility.

Pandora could not continue reading as the tears completely blurred her vision. She tried to wipe them away, but they were a silent flood tide not to be checked. She sat down on one of the chairs and stared blankly at the verdant surroundings, but already they appeared to have lost something. Some stroke of Nature's beauty had been withdrawn. What she had seen before was no longer the same.

Under these distant circumstances, I feel compelled to communicate to you with frankness about the future.

I think it is time to see and accept fully that there will not be a Republic of Colombia, with my father as its leader, and that the dream of your revelation there as the world's first woman doctor is shattered. Perhaps these are indelicate things to say to you at present, but I believe there is a hidden blessing for us both in my father's tragic passing. It suggests a way for you to end of your unnatural deception and for me to be able again to express to you my deep and long-standing love.

My dearest dear, I long for you to return to England and to me where at present I can comfort and care for you. But my wildest hopes travel even further, they dwell on our future together, where I pray you will consent to share life with me as my wife.

No doubt this might seem to you an ordinary existence, void of the intoxications that come with the challenge of charting nascent ground. But, Pandora, my darling, I believe that in the simplicity of familial life, grows a lustrous flame that is fueled by the beauty of children and the power of love.

This masquerade of yours has run its ill-fated course. It is time to face that with truth and make ready your return to those who wait with warmth and tender love.

Your most loving and obedient,

Leander

She reread the first words again and repeated them to herself soundlessly. She never imagined the world without General Miranda. She never imagined her life without him, and now it had come. She looked for his face among the trees and flowers. The birds squawked noisily at each other in hidden branches, but he was gone; and what had been so lovely and gentle an hour ago now seemed harsh and unfriendly.

Questions and memories began to run pell-mell through her mind. What were her limits now? Should she go on? What should she do about her secret? Only the general could answer all of these questions and he was gone. She tried to think of Leander and their life together. Yes, he was strong and brave, he had accomplished much as a soldier and she loved him. But she realized it now, the general had been the rock, the ground, the roots upon which she'd built her life.

***

"He's like a boil on the end of my nose, that's what he is!" stormed Daniel Dennysen, marching up and back before his friend the colonial secretary's fastidiously ordered desk. "I tell you, everywhere I turn, that queer little weasel is poking his flaming red head where it does not belong." He paused briefly to suck in some air. He pressed his knuckles into his desk with his body weight. "Everything which hummed along without the slightest jolt has gone topsy-turvy since that runt arrived. Why, if he's not causing trouble in my prisons, then he's busy issuing edicts on the treatment of our lepers, or better yet, he's meddling in the business of licensing. Let's face it, he has defeated us both at every turn, and the worst of it all, Plaskett!" He banged his fist on the desk. "That damn fool governor, his footman Captain Cloete and the lot, stand behind everything the miscreant does. I tell you now, there's an unholy and unsavory triumvirate there."

"Bring in some sail, man," cautioned Richard Plaskett, who sat unperturbed behind his desk. "Such excitement might throw you into a seizure and then I'd have no alternative but to send for our local 'miracle man,' Dr. Barry himself."

"That's not amusing in the slightest," Dennysen said. "This situation is no cause for levity, and, frankly, I am surprised at your seeming indifference."

"Not at all, my friend." Plaskett absentmindedly fingered a pile of carefully stacked pages to his left. "The fact is, on the other side of that door, sitting in my anteroom at this very moment, is the answer to the Dr. Barry dilemma, a weapon so deliciously powerful, so delightfully unique, no amount of protection or popularity will save the good doctor."

"Don't be cute with me. I have no time for your games or intrigues. What have you got up your sleeve or in your cloakroom?"

"Oh, you'll see, you'll see right now." Plaskett went to the anteroom door. "Nurse McNamara, would you kindly come in, please?"

CHAPTER NINE

Pandora's gait was bold and broad as she strode into the state house, doffing her cockade hat, securing it, military style, under her arm. The questions and fears which had swamped her spirit right after she received Leander's news had now somehow turned to heated optimism and determination—almost as if General Miranda's still heart had been rekindled in her, coursing her blood with renewed purpose. She was ready to fight, her grief was the fuel, the deplorable conditions in the leper colony her fire, and General Miranda was her guardian angel. What better a way, indeed her only way, to be close to him and do him honor.

Lord Somerset's youthful secretary snapped to uneasily as Pandora announced herself loud and clear, with none of the casual repartee he had grown accustomed to on her frequent visits to his lordship.

"They are inside waiting, Dr. Barry sir," he said, blushing, accentuating his platinum hair.

"I apologize for my lateness, gentlemen." Pandora slapped her folio on the long oak table around which her panel was seated. All the old power was present, the elite of Cape Colony, the ruddy-faced Dutch merchants and farmers, the well-fed clergy, smooth-handed board members, and the newly arrived, crisply formal Brits sat eyeing her, side by side, in their own uneasy truce.

But two chairs were empty, the very two she had planned to play to. Lord Plaskett and Mr. Dennysen were conspicuously absent. An uneasiness rattled some of her confidence. They had to be up to something, but she had no time to speculate on what.

"Lord Somerset," she addressed the governor, who sat just to her right. "Gentlemen. Being chief medical officer of the Cape

Colony, I am as you know responsible for the well-being of all its inhabitants, whether they be the Dutch, the British, the Negroes, or Hottentots. This has caused me to ask myself an important question, and I put that question to you now. What gentlemen, are we doing here on this African continent, and what legacy are we to leave?

"We are supposedly civilized men, the elite, if you will. And in our charge we have those who serve us, those humbler than we. The world is changing and the change is in our hands and those who have served us well, those whom we have needed to work our land, care for our crops and prepare our meals, must be looked after. Without them our fortunes would be harder, perhaps impossible to earn. And yet, when some of them have turned ill from the ancient and debilitating disease of leprosy, we have turned our backs on them with cold indifference.

"The Bible says to remove the sufferers from the camp so we are in no danger of contagion, but does it say to shun them? I, gentlemen, have seen these shunned, their broken bodies, their ulcerated, oozing sores, their shredded clothing, their filthy bedding, their insufficient food and water, and I demand it be corrected or it will be on our heads. It will be our legacy that we have cared not for those who had cared for us, that we were unwilling to hear. We were unwilling to do, we were unwilling to show our humanity."

The door opened and three figures appeared. Pandora looked with the others toward the intrusion. There stood the missing Plaskett and Dennysen and between them, her nurse's uniform impeccably starched, was Nurse McNamara. Pandora felt her courage vanish, her mouth suddenly go dry, her temples press in.

"Please excuse the abrupt interruption, Dr. Barry," Lord Plaskett said. "Do continue."

"Lord Plaskett," Cloete stood. "Who is this woman, and why have you brought her into this meeting?"

"Lord Somerset," Plaskett said, now only directing himself to the Governor. "I do beg you forgive my unorthodox entry, but my reason for bringing this woman is of a rather unorthodox and sensitive nature in itself. This woman, sir, is Nurse McNamara, who assisted Dr. Barry with the now famous Caesarian delivery of Mrs.

Munnik. It seems there is some information concerning that night of a highly sensitive nature that the good nurse has until recently kept to herself. But as she is a woman of conscience, she saw fit to impart her secret to me, and I believe it must be passed on."

Pandora wanted to lunge at Plaskett's throat with her hands and tear out his voice. She was frozen to his face despite the excruciating urge and the horrifying inescapability of her situation.

"Lord Plaskett!" Somerset rose. "With such dramatics, let us not wait any further. Please go on."

Playing his hand for all it was worth, Plaskett slowly turned to face Pandora with a look of sickening benevolence washing his expression. "I think, sir, given the delicacy of this matter, it would be far more appropriate if we retired to your private chambers."

"Lord Plaskett, if this is a matter so paramount as to cause your intrusion, I suggest we get on with it at once or I will ask that it rest until tomorrow, when I can give it my full attention." Lord Somerset said.

"Excellency, it is just as you say but I beg that it be conveyed in an appropriate setting and for certain ears alone." Plaskett said a bit of starch taken from his sail.

"Sir, my patience is waning. I have other matters to attend to and too much of the day has already eluded me. I suggest again that we discuss the matter at once or drop it until tomorrow. It appears to me by your argumentativeness that perhaps we can wait until then."

***

Pandora's mind had not stopped churning since she had departed the state house. Cloete had come by to inquire about the mystery and rather than send him away, she had sat with him during supper playing the uncomprehending fool to his "what are they up to, now" questions. She felt more and more trapped by her disguise than ever before. The seriousness of consequence had finally begun to sink in. No more did the challenge of outwitting the curious or insulting them stimulate her battling spirit. She had stepped into the big world and found that she was vulnerable to it, that those who saw her as an enemy would not give way to admiration, but would search for her Achilles heel. And she had one that could not only bring her down but also tumble Cloete and Somerset, who had been her champions and knew nothing of her deception. She could not risk their humiliation just to prove, in this case anyway, that she was upholding a moral and ethical truth against a pair of greedy men fighting for their own self-interests. As much as she hated losing a fight, she accepted that this one was to the conqueror.

Psyche trotted cheerfully along at her heels as she wandered up and down the dark streets, ruminating in the pleasant evening air. She would miss this pioneer place and its strange beauty and way of life, but Leander had been all too wise when he told her that deceptions only breed more deceptions, and even before his letter and today's events, she had begun to have mixed feelings about going on with her choice.

Despite the second-naturedness of her life as James Barry, she had begun to tire of the constant pressure that discovery might happen. The misery and suffering of the lepers and others here, though all that she had trained for and full of purpose, had become an exhausting grind with little respite. She could not form a real attachment to anyone. Cloete, her dearest friend, really knew nothing of her at all and as her feelings toward him had grown into a true friendship, the more vulgar she found her secret. The others, the Somerset girls and Mr. and Mrs. Munnik, provided great pleasure for her but still she must always keep one eye on the deception, to make sure there was no exposure to light. How perfect now that on the very eve of her discovery she should be walking along in the darkness with only her frisky dog by her side.

Leander still waited for her. She was ready to admit he was right. And yes, she loved him, as she knew, despite her ways, he still loved her. Why then keep to this madness when there was a fine and noble alternative? Surprisingly she found herself standing before Nurse McNamara's rooming house. The moon sneaked in and out of the clouds, lighting and dimming the little flower boxes in the windows. Without hesitation, as she had obviously been heading here all along, she pulled Mrs. Van Roebuch, the charwoman's bell.

"Dr. Barry!" the woman said, opening the door. "Is anything

wrong?"

"Not terribly, Madame, but I would like to speak with Nurse McNamara if I may."

"Yes, of course, I believe she is in, I did not hear her go out. Take this light and follow the hall at the top of the stair."

Pandora knocked two or three times on the door to no response and was about to return downstairs, when Psyche, who had been scratching on the door, pushed it open, its latch apparently not quite closed. When her light penetrated the dark, Pandora saw Nurse McNamara sprawled across her bed, her hair unclipped and in disarray, her slips helter-skelter and her arm dangling down the side of the bed with an empty glass beneath it on the floor. On the bedside table stood a half-empty bottle of gin. Pandora stepped close enough to see the puffy face, which stared up only half aware of her intruders. It was clear she was totally inebriated. For a moment Pandora just stood, there letting light spilling across the disheveled woman.

"My God! It's you, what? Please, get out." The nurse shot up straight, unconsciously fumbling with her buttons and skirts. Her hair fell in her face and stuck on the perspiration spots that had formed on her brow and neck. "You have no business, have no right, you can't just barge in—uh, I am ill with a toothache," she said, seeing Pandora looking at the bottle.

"It's all right, nurse," Pandora said. "I am not here to threaten you or spy or report your condition. I am not going to blackmail you. I am merely here because I think we should have a talk. Woman to woman."

CHAPTER TEN

The strong sun hitting the side of the state house shone harshly into Governor Somerset's office. Cloete drew the shears across the windows, softening the glare. Plaskett, Dennysen and Nurse McNamara sat uneasily watching the door.

Lord Somerset looked at the large wall clock, which ticked monotonously on towards three o'clock. "Well, gentlemen, Nurse McNamara, in ten minutes we will have waited a half-hour for the doctor. I suggest we abandon our vigil and proceed with whatever this business is before I lose my patience, or we all lose any more valuable time to the matter."

"I've sent Secretary Farnsworth to the doctor's quarters," Cloete said. "Perhaps an emergency arose and detained him."

"Or it could be something else," Plaskett said, evoking a cat who ate the bird smile from Mr. Dennysen.

"What's your meaning, sir?" Cloete snapped.

"Fear of the truth, I would assume," said Plaskett.

"All right, gentlemen, enough parrying. Have the nurse swear the truth, and let's get on with it, Dr. Barry or not," said Governor Somerset.

Cloete held the Bible to Nurse McNamara, who swore to the truth with a strong forthrightness.

"Lord Plaskett," the governor said, "you may speak first, since this whole event has been at your request."

"Thank you Lord Somerset, I am grateful for the opportunity to expose an unthinkable and heinous situation, which could destroy—"

"Lord Plaskett, we do not need a political dissertation right now. We simply need you to state your charge."

"I am sorry sir, my enthusiasm in putting a quick end to this ugly matter, as Lord Fiscal, I feel it only – "

"Thank you," said Somerset.

"Of course, yes, well. It was brought to my attention by the good-willed testimony of Nurse McNamara, that Dr. Barry, our chief medical examiner, is not at all what we think him to be. It seems that on the night that Dr. Barry performed the ungodly surgery on Mrs. Munnik – which I say only through Providence was a success – the good nurse, having reason found it necessary to seek Dr. Barry in his guest room at the Munnik home. I would ask that Nurse McNamara continue from here as to what she encountered upon that visit."

"Very well, Nurse McNamara," Somerset said.

"Well, your Lordship, it was really not much of anything. I knocked upon Dr. Barry's door and when I got no response for some minute or two I quietly allowed myself in. As the proceedings of the evening had been quite taxing, the doctor was sound asleep, a book upon his chest, his boots still on. When he became aware of my presence, he was naturally startled, not remembering where he was and all, and I must say, he dressed me down quite sharply."

"Go on to what is important, woman," Plaskett said.

"Sirs, that is really all there is to it. I stated my apology and my reason for the intrusion. The doctor dismissed me and I departed."

"My good nurse!" Plaskett went and stood nervously by the window, spreading his legs and stiffening his posture. "Did you not tell me that when you entered Dr. Barry's room he was in a rather complete state of undress, and much to your shock and honor, you saw clearly that Dr. Barry was not a man at all, but a woman? Did you not tell me that!"

Dennysen giggled at the excitement, and both Cloete and Lord Somerset turned a keen attention to the proceedings.

"Well, Nurse McNamara," Somerset said, "did you tell Lord Plaskett such a thing?"

"Yes sir, Lord Governor. I did tell him that, but it was a lie."

"A lie! A wha – ? Imposs – ? Wha – !"

"Calm yourself, Plaskett," Somerset said. "Go on, Nurse McNarnara."

"Well you see, sir, it had been a very hard day and I was not at all in favor of the doctor's methods. So that when he succeeded and the beautiful child came so well and all turned out, I was a good bit put off. Then, when later he was so unkind to me for intruding, and as it is I have a lonely life that leads me to a bit too much drink at times, well, sir, I only acted out of malice and vindictiveness. The truth is I have come to know that Dr. Barry is an exceptional person and great surgeon. My own small nature could not accept that at first—and so, having heard the talk about the doctor's duel with Mr. Cloete, I created this horrible lie. But I only thought it would fuel some gossip and then go away. I was wrong, and I apologize to you, I only wish I could make it right with Dr. Barry, who is truly the most unique and exceptional person I have ever met. I have come to realize he deserves all our respect and admiration."

"Well, Lord Fiscal, there seems to be quite a breach here. It is now obvious you have no charges or scandalous news for me at all regarding Dr. Barry. Therefore I see no reason to pursue the matter. I will say, though, not knowing whether your motives are biased, I do not admire the zealousness with which you attempted to produce a scandal. It is far from gentlemanly and far from English. We are not at Cape Colony to undermine ourselves or those in our govern. As a lesson to you, I am appointing you in charge of the leper colony at Hemel-ard. You will see to it that the reforms Dr. Barry requested are implemented to the letter, as I have seen fit to accept them."

***

The clock chimed the half hour. The sun had moved away from the window. Cloete opened the curtains and watched a diminishing ship leave the harbor.

On deck, Pandora and Psyche watched the land disappear.

"Dr. Barry, your bags are unpacked, and I've served tea in your cabin. I can bring it to you here if you prefer," said the steward.

"Yes, I would, thank you."

Pandora sat in a deck chair in the shade. Psyche jumped into her lap, chipper and enthusiastic about a new adventure. "Yes, Psyche," she held his earnest face steady, his black eyes looking straight at her. "We're going home," she said.

CHAPTER ELEVEN

The carriage came to a slow stop in front of 10 Grafton Street. The driver lay the reins of the horses down, and Pandora rose and stood on the lip, before the driver could alight and assist. She was wearing her blue dress uniform and, with what had become a kind of trademark, she flourished the removal of her broad cockade hat. "Stay seated," she said to her driver, "and keep Psyche with you. I will either be making a brief visit, or someone will come to fetch my bags." Psyche sat alert, his little tongue hanging out, his energy anticipating her beckoning. "No, Psyche, stay," Pandora said. Sadly, the dog returned to his belly and knitted his brow at her.

Pandora pushed open the gate and entered the courtyard with the grand old sycamore. The cobbled court seemed unchanged. She looked at the familiar bumpy ground littered with the twigs and leaves of the trees, fallen there after so many rainy and windy seasons. The flower boxes were bright and merry with Sarah's perfect touch, and the windows were shiny clean behind them. Somehow Pandora had expected even the stones to appear in a state of mourning in deference to Miranda's passing. But she should have remembered that this was a hearty and stolid household, which adjusted to the extraordinary. Of course things looked polished and bright, perhaps just a bit smaller, more contained than her memory had made them.

Sarah was sitting on a lawn chair, facing the great honeysuckle bush that crawled lavishly over the back wall. The sweet smell its blooms produced coated the air. Pandora couldn't see whether she was asleep or not, but she crept behind her and clamped her gloved hands over the woman's eyes.

"What! Oh, my! Who is this?" Sarah took hold of the hands which had momentarily darkened her light.

"You'll 'ave te make a guess, mum," Pandora said. Sarah took away Pandora's hands and looked questioningly at the uniformed figure above her. Her face was still soft and lovely, but a greyness had washed over it all. The mantle of loss and grieving had left her undeniably changed.

"Pandora, my good God! I didn't recognize you – oh my!" She grabbed Pandora's shoulders and enveloped her in her arms. Pandora could feel her body heave gently with the tears and sobs that rose freely. "My blessed child, you're home at last."

The two held each other, Pandora allowing long buried feelings of familial love and care to seep from Sarah's being into hers and back again. They said nothing, there was no need, everything was in their embrace.

"Leander, Topham, Carmen! Look who's returned! Come, come." Sarah took Pandora's hand and pulled her towards the house. "Come see who's here," she called again, till Topham appeared pushing his wheelbarrow from around the other side of the house.

"My lord Jesus!" he bellowed, grabbing Pandora in his bear arms and swinging her once around. The upstairs window flew open, and Carmen let out a shriek as she saw Pandora. Then the front door opened, and Leander stepped onto the little top step and stood still. Pandora faced him, a feeling of embarrassment and timidity overtaking her.

His features had darkened and become powerful without being hard. A saber scar streaked from his ear to his jaw. Even in civilian clothes he stood like a soldier, and the pride of his duty issued from every part of him. "I don't know whether to salute or kiss you," he said. Pandora felt a weakness behind her knees and one of her uncontrollable laughs begin to percolate.

"Don't be a donkey, Major, I didn't come halfway around the world for smart remarks."

He nearly knocked her over before she felt her feet leave the ground and his warm lips met hers. She lost all shame in that moment. She was glad to be home.

***

Everything for the dinner was prepared. As always, the table had fresh flowers, candles were lit, the food abundant. Carmen, now without Rosa, who had run off with a boxer named Lopes, bustled about. Her cheeks were scarlet from her hasty preparations in the overly hot kitchen. The fire roared and the good old reliable rain had obliterated the bit of sun that had vainly tried to ring out the day. Everyone was settled in his rightful place. General Miranda's chair had been moved permanently to a place against the wall. Leander sat at the head now in his own special chair. Despite the small gathering, there was much conviviality. Topham sang some silly old tunes. Carmen shrieked with laughter and wept unmercifully at Leander's stories of drunken escapades in the Portuguese campaign and his touching salute to the memory of his father. Sarah listened, her face brightened with love when the general's name arose, and some of the grey shroud that seemed her veil parted with the sweetness that the evening brought. Pandora recounted only one story, that of her duel. The good food, the cozy warmth inside her home, and the embrace of her family had made her very tired.

"Pandora dear, I don't wish to interject a touchy subject, but what are your plans for the future? Are you going to continue as an army doctor now that the general has gone and the—" tears cut off the rest of Sarah's query.

"I think, right off, I'll get a good night's sleep," she said. "Then tomorrow I'm going to start thinking about what to do with my hair." Everyone laughed.

But she was not at all happy at the way her close-cropped hair looked when she had donned one of her lovely dresses. She remembered how much she had liked all her floppy curls which complemented the colorful clothes she'd always chosen. This army look was not going to do.

"Excuse me a moment," Leander said over the laughter. "But you are absent without leave, are you not?"

"Indeed, Major, I am. Are you going to turn me in?"

"Ole, touché!" Carmen and Topham heckled.

"I think tomorrow will be time enough to discuss the military status of Staff Surgeon Barry. But right now I am going to turn myself in to my cozy bed and listen to the rain." Pandora rose, kissed Sarah and the others. "Come sit with me a moment in the library, Leander. You can impress me with how correct and brave you are."

They hadn't gone two steps along the gallery when Leander took her hand. His assertiveness thrilled and relieved her. So long had she been her own assertive force, so often pushing too hard not to show any chink in her armor. Now she could let go and parry when she wanted, and succumb when she didn't—all a woman's prerogative.

"All right," Leander said, walking between her and the big fireplace in the library, the lively flames behind him emphasizing his tall, dark silhouette. "Did you come back to marry me or not?"

Pandora had hoped for a touch of romance in their old rendezvous before they took up serious matters. But any fears she may have had about his feelings towards her, now that she was here in the flesh, fled upon his directness.

"We certainly are straight up front," she said. "But I should have thought a kiss or at the very least a bent knee were due prior to such a question."

"Don't play with me now, Pandora. I've asked a question."

"Do you still love me?" she teased.

"I love you more than my own life." Leander stood in the exact middle of the mantle, his whole figure framed by firelight.

"You're not disappointed to see me unattractive and older?"

"My God, you're surely no less damnable than ever."

She laughed and jumped back into the game. "Leander, you would think two old soldiers like us could indulge in one night of uncomplicated romance, after all these years of duty, responsibility and faithfulness." She looked slyly at him. "I most certainly have been true to you. Dare I ask you the same?"

Leander's broad smile was rich with innuendo.

"You blackguard, you common whoremonger. And you're going to lecture me about honor!"

"Wait one moment, dear lady. You never gave me your promise!"

"Good night, sir!" She rushed to the stair.

"Pandora, you can't be jeal—"

"Filthy philanderer!"

Leander grabbed the bottom of her skirt just as she crossed the top rung. She kicked herself free.

"Don't you dare chase me or come near me." She turned to slam her door on him, but he was already half in. He pushed her onto her bed. "Get out, you dog, you're a dog."

"Shut up!" Leander kissed her, and the warmth of his mouth made all her feelings of jealousy vanish. All she felt was an uninhibited passion charging through her as his body lay over her.

"What are you going to do, challenge me to a duel?" he asked, rolling on his back. "And don't think I didn't notice the twinkle in your eye when Captain Cloete's name was spoken."

"Preposterous! I was a man, remember?"

Leander reached under her and brought her to him. "You're not a man now, and I want you to answer my question."

"Yes, I will marry you, Leander. I love you."

CHAPTER TWELVE

Pandora's mind treaded through troubling doubts as their fiacre rounded the corner of Rue d'Italien and she looked with wonder at a Paris considerably changed from the one she knew. The Great Emperor had come and gone, but his mark was everywhere. The fiacre wended its way past the yet completed church of St. Madeline. Pandora fanned herself briskly, for the August sun beat down on their carriage and the closeness inside stifled the air. But as they passed the Opera Comique and turned onto the open boulevard, a breeze found its way inside.

Pandora lay her fan again in her lap and leaned back. Closing her eyes, she remembered the dark city of her youth, so different from the cosmopolitan sophistication which twinkled around her now. Gone were the marauding gangs of bizarre incroyables and the bloodthirsty sans coulottes, the shuttered houses, the air full of fear, and the street children unkempt and uncared-for in every district. Paris's old scars were now masked with new construction and though much remained unfinished, the promise of improvement was evidenced everywhere. She breathed deeply the grass-fresh air as they left the close quarters of the inner city and entered the outskirts. Seeing all this, Pandora tried to imagine how the years and their events must have changed Mademoiselle Peliciàn.

"You know, Pandora," Leander said, sensing as two lovers do, the other's thoughts." She may have moved or passed on."

"No, she is alive and here," Pandora said, turning to him and taking both his hands in hers. Their wedding rings looked so shiny and new on their fingers. "I know she is alive. It is not some whim or wish, and I cannot rationally defend it, but believe me, I know she is alive."

"Well, just as you know she is alive," Leander said, "somehow I know she is well and in good spirits."

"Well then, we are a confident union of irrationality," Pandora said. "In my opinion that is the best kind."

At last they turned onto Rue Menilmontant and stopped sharply in front of number seventeen. "We're here!" Pandora said, starting out of the cab. She ran to the steps of the house, looking quickly around at the surroundings. At least this block had not changed very much, though the shutters of her house had gone from lemon yellow to a fresh coat of blue. Charged by their arrival, Pandora quickly lifted the lion's tongue and knocked three times. She waited an appropriate span although she thought herself too patient, then knocked again. Still no sound from inside, her fear that maybe Mademoiselle had passed on, cracking both her and Leander's hopeful irrationality. She put her ear to the door but heard no noise behind it. "There is no one here!" She came back to Leander, who was waiting just beside the carriage.

"Well, someone must live here, why don't we come back later after tea." Leander took her arm to help her back in but as she stepped up she saw through the other side of the carriage, a big woman laden with packages coming across the street.

"Leander," she whispered, "that's her crossing our way." She peeked out the back as Mademoiselle reached the curb. "Yes, it's Mademoiselle, she's coming. Now don't say a word, don't let on a thing. Let me do all the talking, just follow what I do and say."

"May I help you?" Mademoiselle squinted coarsely at the two.

"Oh my, well, yes indeed, I believe you might," Pandora said, with an overly-stuffed Englishness. "You'll pardon, I meant to ask, is this number seventeen Menilmontant?"

"Yes, madame, it is, do you have business here?"

"Do you speak English?" Pandora asked.

"Not a single word. Don't need it, don't like it. Now what's your business, Madame? It's hot and I'm tired and don't have time to chat with you."

"My business, yes, well, we have just arrived from London and a friend said we might find a Mademoiselle Peliciàn at this address. That she, being a good cook and housekeeper, might be engaged if the price were right."

"I am Mademoiselle Peliciàn. Who is it in London who referred you?" Mademoiselle's face suddenly had lit up with such an expression of hope. Pandora couldn't keep up her ruse any longer. She wrested the woman's packages from her.

"Mademoiselle, do you not recognize, even faintly, the face of a small girl whom you bathed and fed and whose mass of red curls you cursed and tugged until they fell freely about a sparkling clean face? Do you not see a trace of a wild urchin whom you cajoled and scolded until she turned to a creature of civility? Do you not see a touch of the child to whom you bid farewell under the cloak of night after placing a black box into her adoring hand," Pandora implored, offering over the battered tin.

"Mon Dieu!" the woman shrieked, slamming her huge, work-worn fingers into her mouth. "Can it be? Is it really possible? Have my prayers been answered?" she cried up to the sky, which became the receiver of her exhortations.. "Heaven be praised! Praise to God and to Thy glory! My child has returned to me before I close my eyes forever! Thank you, sweet Jesus in Heaven!"

In one sweeping movement, Mademoiselle Peliciàn buried Pandora into her arms, their tears landing together on her cushiony breasts as the old woman clutched her close like a bear, never again to part from its cub.

After a little while, Pandora took Mademoiselle Peliciàn by the hand and extended the other to Leander. "Yes, Mademoiselle, it is, I and this fine man is my husband, Major Miranda, the son of our general."

CHAPTER THIRTEEN

"Now, don't worry, Leander, I only plan on buying a shawl for Mademoiselle Peliciàn, and then I'm just going to look around," she said, while Leander paid their cab fare. But the feast at the Palais Royal was too much for her, and she dragged Leander from shop to shop where even he lost his materialistic reserve. He allowed himself to be convinced that gaiters were definitely in order, along with a silk cravat, a white hat, a shillelagh and a box of expensive cigars.

They rested briefly in the enclosed garden. Then Pandora blazed a trail down the gravel path overhung with orange trees, bowers of camilia, fleur-de-lis and Bengal rose, after their tantalizing fragrances restored her drive. At a perfumer she purchased a small iris cologne for Leander, while he, on the second tier of the parallelogrammed mall, found a bookseller and bought a finely bound Moliere. Having covered nearly the full half-mile of the piazza, up one side and down the other, Leander had had enough for one day. He found a small resting place and delved into his new purchase while the tireless Pandora rushed on to complete the distance.

"The classics are classics precisely because they have endured fools such as yourself," said a double-chinned patrician, the jacket over his rounded belly spotted with food stains. "They have weathered puny insults in the past and will no doubt have to weather them again." He rocked forward on his toes, while the long sparse wisps of smoke which encircled his too-small head floated randomly as he attacked his listener.

"It is a new age, I tell you!" his equally half-sized partner retaliated, putting a finger into the other's middle. "A new glory for

France, growing above the horizon of the past. These new Romantic writers will bring all—not just the effete—back to art with a real sense of life, not the paper thin whinings and whimperings of that old bankrupt upper strata."

Leander quickly took interest in this debate and slid close enough to draw away their attention.

"Well, what do you have to say?" the first small man demanded, startling Leander.

"Oh, well, sir," he stood up abruptly, having already begun to compose his reply. "I must decline an opinion in this matter, as I am only a guest in your fine city and do not think it fitting for a foreigner to take sides in such a deeply felt conflict."

"But not at all! Do give us your opinion," the two men encouraged.

"Well, if I may be so bold as to venture an uninformed but diplomatic opinion, perhaps you may use it to see past your stalemate. I would say that if the future of France's literary arts is to match the glory of its past, then neither of you have cause for concern. You see, only the finest flower can burst forth from soil raked and hoed by Corneille, Racine, and Moliere. So, gentlemen, please don't waste your gifts on acrimonious debate when clearly a call for celebration and unity is in order."

"Well done!" grinned the Modernist, with a warm expression. His head of well-oiled thick black hair vibrating up and down in agreement. "Leave it to an Englishman to safely navigate a perfect course through tricky waters."

"My thanks to you, as well, for the compliment, sir," Leander said, relaxing his shoulders which he realized were lifted rather stiffly. "Since you have inquired after my opinion, I feel it is only fit to turn the tables around and ask after yours."

"We are at your service," bowed the double chin.

"Our minds are joined to your favor," chirped the nattily oiled one, not to be outdone.

"Let us assume," Leander began, summoning a tone of temptation, "that either of you gentlemen were married to the most beautiful and beguiling woman in the world, where would you choose to dine with her, given this glorious city so full of culinary choices?"

"Ah! Delighted!" burst the smaller fellow, fulfilling a graceful relevé. "This is the most serious, yet engaging proposition set forth to me in quite some time and, I will venture to say, even mon ami Paul will agree when I insist that Les Trois Freres Provencal is the only possibility."

"Absolutment, sans doute, c'est incroyable et parfait," jumped in Paul, kissing his fingers to the heavens. "Mon ami Armand is one hundred percent correct. We are in total accord that Les Trois Freres is the finest of the fine restaurants in Paris and certainly equal to the most beautiful of women!"

"Of course, one must order the cutlets with cheese..." Armand broke in.

"Cutlets with cheese!" shouted Paul, blanching at the thought. "Ahaha! Who is the peasant now? Everyone knows that one cannot dine at Les Trois without savoring the delectable duck."

"You are an imbecile—a true Corsican!" Armand reddened. "I do not know why on earth I allow myself to accept your association. Duck is so common a dish that it only pleases the most uninitiated palate."

"Cutlets and cheese," bellowed Paul, shaking his finger in the air, "I feed to my dog!"

Just then, and much to his relief, Leander spied Pandora coming their way carrying several small packages. He watched her from a distance. Her bright face, trademark curls (nearly their full length again), and her slim graceful figure made him admit to himself that he had not boasted—she was indeed the most beautiful woman in the world.

***

"I really don't know why you insisted we come here. I had so wanted to go to Verys." Pandora's forehead wrinkled and her eyes gave a pouty expression as she tried to muster some real vexation at Leander's choice of restaurant.

"Why Pandora, you are not aware that at present Les Trois Freres is the absolutment de Paris? That all the most sophisticated and enlightened of Paris dine here? My goodness, I thought you were very in the know. This just proves once again how deceived one can be about another, especially if one is madly in love." Leander reached under the table and squeezed Pandora's knee in that most sensitive spot.

"Ach!" she laughed grabbing his hand. "When did you become such a lover of fine cuisine? Or should I ask, who taught you these subtle virtues?"

"Play fair, Pandora," Leander said. "I had hoped by bringing you to the finest French restaurants you might learn some culinary secrets and thus be able to reproduce the excellent meals when we have settled at home. I doubt whether your years in South Africa prepared you for the rigors of domestic life."

"Now who should play fairly?"

"I'm sorry, darling, it's just that these two impossibly Parisian characters..."

"Pardon, monsieur et madame." A very erect, tight-upper-lipid waiter commanded attention. "You have decided?" His tone of disdain made Pandora cover her face with her menu as she could not stifle a broad grin.

"What do you recommend?" she said, from behind her screen.

"Well, Madame, most of the strangers prefer the cutlets and cheese," the waiter said, his contempt spilling all over the table.

"Cutlets and cheese!" Leander said, loud enough to raise the arrogant garcon's eyebrows. "Good fellow, cutlets and cheese is what we English feed to our dogs."

"But of course, pardon, excuse me." The waiter squirmed and looked about to see if other patrons were staring at them. "Perhaps Madame would enjoy a delicate roast duck,"

"Duck indeed!" Leander struck the table with his menu. "Are you implying that Madame has plebian tastes?" Now others were gaping at their commotion. "Monsieur et Madame will first sample the bouille, then bring us your mourue d'ail along with French beans, broccoli, and a bottle of your finest Bouchet."

"Excellent, monsieur, excellent!" The waiter bowed effusively, nearly falling over the neighboring table as he made for the kitchen.

"And now, madame, what was it we were discussing?" Leander winked at Pandora.

"I am quite impressed," she said.

***

When they exited the restaurant a rain had left the streets damp and fresh, but looking up they saw that whatever had fallen, the cloud which had brought it was now passed and the sky was starlit and clear.

"Now it's my turn to take charge," Pandora said, leading Leander across the Rue de Chartres toward the Théatre de Vaudeville. They had to pause for a moment as the trebling of the military police heralded preparations for their watch. High-stepping and high-hatted, the military police came down the street, crossed ammunition belts gleaming even in the dim light. Once in the square they broke into ever diminishing groups, going off in unison to their patrols until only the drummer and signal man were left. "We'll get a fiacre just across there by the theater," Pandora said, darting ahead of Leander, calling to the one in front whose driver was as old as Methuselah and as thin as he was ancient. "Pont Neuf," Pandora said as Leander helped her inside the cab.

The narrow streets were crammed with people, and the driver had to maneuver carefully. Light spilled out from open doorways and half-shuttered windows. Snatches of chatter, dickering and gaiety flooded out like the light. Leander and Pandora sat quietly absorbing it all.

"We'll walk from here!" Pandora said, rapping on the carriage top. "The bridge is right over there." She pointed to it and darted into the crowd. Leander lagged to pay the fare. "Well, that's new." Pandora pointed to a statue of Henry IV erected at the opposite side of the bridge.

"What did you say?" Leander puffed.

"I said that statue, oh, Leander," she said, stepping onto the bridge and taking his arm. "This is where we begin. This is the Paris not written of in the guide books or spoken of in fancy parlors. This is where I began my life."

Before taking another step, she stood holding her husband's arm and stared at the circus-like bustle that stretched across the Pont Neuf between the two banks of the city. It hadn't had this atmosphere in her years here, though life and livelihood had gone on atop and below. "Onward!" she said, sallying forth with a schoolgirl's enthusiasm. An old artisan was deftly putting the finishing touches of green paint on the thread-thin chutes of an orange tree sculpture. He looked up at them and smiled from under his tobacco-stained mustache as they stopped to watch him.

"A fine evening, monsieur et madame."

"Indeed so," Leander said, dropping a coin in the man's box.

"Attend," he said, handing Leander a small palm sized orange all woven and twined with wire and painted with loving care. "Pour madame," he pointed to Pandora who was way ahead, watching two buskers toss flaming pins back and forth in a dangerously high arc. Leander pulled her a little out of their path as he sensed she was too agitated to exercise caution.

A pair of acrobats caused their necks to strain, as one performed a handstand from the feet of the other who was in a headstand atop two dozen or so books. A fat woman with bright blond curls sat on an old washtub playing the hurdy-gurdy. Then they came to a group of Ethiopian serenaders, singing strange Eastern tunes, their bright, loose shirts and high hats quite different from the norm.

"May God strike me dead if this miraculous elixir will not grow hair on an egg," shouted a man wearing tight striped pants, standing atop a box by the edge of the bridge. "If you want to preserve your youthful look forever, a refreshing massage of just a few drops of this scientific marvel will do the trick. I personally guarantee it."

Leander paused to listen. "Come along," Pandora tugged.

"I thought you might want me to buy you some of that," Leander said, taking her in his arms.

"I don't need it."

"Not now, but someday," he said.

Pandora pushed him away and just near the end of the bridge she took a hurdle to the dark embankment below. "Stay close and mind your step," she hollered up to Leander, as she jackrabbited down a secret path littered with bottles, pieces of clothing, and odd shoes, the remnants of many a rough encounter. "The tour begins here." Pandora spread her arms, embracing the whole of this dark, dank, mystery-laden spot. Leander slid uncomfortably down to join her on the quay. "This was my Paris."

From under the bridge came a rattle of loose stones. They could not make out a figure in the smoke pot thickness of the underlying air, but then a humpback dwarf appeared and smiled toothlessly with false humility.

"A good night to you monsieur et madame. May I help you find your way?"

"No need, my friend," Leander stepped in front of Pandora and quickly dropped a coin in the tramp's hat, making sure the man knew he was both big and unafraid. "We are exactly where we intend to be."

"Then I bid you good night again," the dwarf said, half crawling like a crab up the embankment and disappearing onto the bridge.

"I used to hide my money over there," she pointed to the bricks half buried under part of the bridge. "There are still loose ones," she said, coming away and looking into the dark Seine. "I can almost see my own dirty face and matted hair, when I catch my reflection. It's so long ago and so much has happened. It seems like it wasn't my life at all, but someone else's." Pandora threw a pebble, rippling the water. "Shall we erase the slate and go forward?"

"No. Let us fill it and build one life out of it," Leander said, as they again returned to the street.

Pandora led them through narrow alleys and up twisting streets lined with bent houses of odd shapes, which cast shadows like old men buttressed by their crooked canes. As they passed two hawk-eyed dustmen who stood smoking in the spill-light of a half-open doorway, one of them spit in their general direction. "They certainly don't look pleased to see us," Leander said.

"Our kind do not pass this way very often, and when they do it arouses contempt," Pandora said, coldly, then turned onto a lighted lane full of tumult. "This is the pet-au-diable," she said. Leander did his best to keep up, bobbing and weaving his way through the pushcart barkers. The smells of Oriental fragrances filled his nose while strange tongues clacked exotic rhythms into his ears. "This is the section of the Jews!"

Pandora stopped in front of an armoire-sized dry goods store packed with shoeless children. "You see that man over there," she said, pointing to a frail stationer whose cart stood first in the row, its proprietor wearing fingerless gloves in open defiance of the summer season. "Each night while your father was in prison, I would buy writing paper from that man."

Without another word she led Leander away, expertly negotiating them backwards and tiptoeing over the muddy ruts in her satin slippers until they came onto an esplanade. It curved in accord with a filthy kennel, which carried its fetid dross down the middle. They threaded around corners blocked by gatherings of gamblers and passed numerous palaces of iniquity whose coarse, harsh noises carried into the street a measure of peril.

"Flower, miss? Buy your lady a flower, sir?" hawked the strong voice of a little girl, who appeared to Pandora to be no more than six years. She stood directly in their path underneath a flickering lamp which lit the sign of the Pigeon Breast Tavern. Her once-blue smock, now faded to gray, was worn thin at the shoulders and printed with muck. In one hand she extended a small, battered bunch of buttercups with their heads drooping and their color washed out, like her dress. With the other hand she clutched the baby fingers of a heavy-lidded boy whose eyes kept drifting shut and whose pudgy legs were buckling under him as sleep tried to win him over. But each time he began to near the sodden ground, the girl yanked him upright. His nose was runny, his cheeks were puffy, and his blond hair was tousled and grimy.

"Is he your brother?" Pandora asked.

"Oui, madame, me one and only brother," the girl said, suspiciously eyeing Pandora.

"How much are the flowers?"

"Two for a sous," chirped the girl, simultaneously jerking up her brother's arm.

"Special for you!" the boy blurted, his eyes popping wide, fulfilling his part in the couplet. Pandora knelt down, ignoring the threat of soil on her skirts.

"Did you make that up all by yourself?" she asked, drawing the child to her by the waist.

"Yes, madame, and peoples like it!"

"I'm sure they do," Pandora said, straightening the girl's smock. "How many flowers do you have left, young lady?"

"Just these five." She thrust the tired lot in front of Pandora. "But I'll tell you what. If you buys four, I'll throw the fifth one in free. How's that?" the little gamin said with a wink, cocking her head to one side sealing the proposition.

"Leander, give me a gold Louis, please." Pandora rose, accepted the bouquet, then pressed a large gold coin into the child's hand.

"My god, lady," snapped the girl angrily, "what do you think I am—a banker? Why, it'd take me a double-week to make change for this piece!"

"No change," Pandora said. "That is for you and your brother."

"What's the trick?"

"There is no trick. Just put it in your pocket and don't let anyone take it from you."

In a flash the urchin had snatched her brother and disappeared down the nearest alley. Leander put his arm around Pandora's shoulders and tightened her shawl securely to ward against the damp. They wandered in silence, making their way back to the quay. As the first pink of morning played on the Seine, they sat shoulder to shoulder under the Pont Neuf, watching the old river roll on its way.

"I do so want a baby," Pandora said, at last. Leander slipped the little wire orange into her hand.

CHAPTER FOURTEEN

The cold rain pelted the roof and windows of the house on Rue Menilmontant. Pandora lay still in the bed listening, the big quilts all warm and cozy on top of her. Leander was completely undisturbed by this March torrent and so far baby Francesca seemed unaroused. The birth had been lengthy, but uneventful, and Pandora only felt minor discomfort from its residue. But even this had dimmed not one bit of her joy and elation over the birth of their child. She waited for a sound from the little bassinet; when it came, her milk let down in that miraculous way, producing that tingling sensation. She would go and sit in the rocker with her newborn and, using her foot to push the chair to and fro, she'd watch little Francesca while she fed. She always woke before the baby, but she didn't mind. She would just lie still, thinking about Francesca and picturing her asleep a little distance away.

The baby was born small, but Pandora remembered that even at the first moment of life, she had given such a howl, Leander had rushed into the room in fear. Her little back was straight and firm and she now had a bit of black fuzz atop her head, a sure Miranda trait. Mademoiselle had said she knew from the first that Francesca was of an obstinate spirit, just like her mother.

Pandora smiled to herself. Maybe in the not too distant future she would understand what it had been for Mademoiselle and the general to raise her. This was her only sadness, that General Miranda was not here to see what had come of her union with Leander, that they were happy and well and that he had a grandchild to tell the tales of his adventurous life to while she sat on his knee. Or that he could dream the dreams of the future with another young adventurer.

In late summer they would return to England. Sarah was most impatient to have her grandchild close by and, in the meanwhile, Pandora was smoothing out the wrinkles in her scheme to bring Mademoiselle back with them. Naturally, Mademoiselle had no desire to abandon this comfortable home which the general had left her, nor was she interested in foreign regions. France was just fine for her and the "other grandmother" could come and live with them here. But Pandora had noticed Mademoiselle was beginning to show her years quite markedly and since she had no one left of her family Pandora did not want to leave her alone. Mademoiselle needed to take life more easily and in England people would care for her and of course they would immediately love her as she had been everything to the general when he had been in need in France.

Francesca's fuss drew Pandora from her plans; the milk responded as always. She slipped into her wool slippers, good protection from the cold floor.

"Shh, shh, shh, Mother's coming," she cooed, as she walked to the straw bassinet, now swaying from Francesca's call. "Here I am, my darling child," Pandora sang, but when she reached the bed, Francesca's face was contorted in pain, her skin was a sickening blue. "Leander!" she called, quickly unfastening the soiled diaper. The stool was unusually dark. Pandora looked at it more closely. "My God! Leander!" she screamed. The bowel was thick with black blood.

"What is it! What is the matter!" Leander was at her side in an instant.

"It can't be! No, no!" Pandora held the baby tightly to her breast, cradling the little head in her palm. "Mademoiselle, Mademoiselle!" she screamed, now running towards Peliciàn's room, drawing Francesca's little body ever tighter in her embrace, pressing her head to her neck.

"What is it!" Mademoiselle was already in the doorway of her room. The body in Pandora's arms convulsed just once then went limp, the life fled.

"No! No! No!" Pandora wailed.

***

The two large candles stood like solemn columns on either side of the dead child's cradle. The flames burned hollow excavations deep into their necks, creating a somber, shadowy light, which cast itself onto the still child's waxen cheeks. Pandora stood plumb line straight above the sepulchral cradle. Her dark ringed eyes were open wide, and she stared in wild fixation straight ahead at the smoking incense burner, which was placed on a small table between the two vigil lights. Almost imperceptibly, her fingertips rocked the crib. Its creaking rhythm eerily broke the silence of the stark parlor.

Mademoiselle Peliciàn had removed all of the furniture from the room, save for a few chairs and the cradle. The paintings and mirrors were draped in black and all light except for the votaries was eliminated. The glow of happiness which had so recently returned to this home had been extinguished with crushing grief-laden speed. Pandora's face was drawn and desiccated. Her black clad frame seemed to have been captured by a gauntness that instantly purged what was left of her youth. Mademoiselle sat stationed by the door, her lips praying voicelessly while her fingers traveled her worn beads. Leander sat at the other side of her, his eyes never leaving Pandora for a moment. They were a grieving triangle, Pandora controlling the apex with her absent rocking, Leander and Mademoiselle at the bottom on either side of the closed door.

A sharp knock jolted Leander. He rose and paused only a fraction to measure Pandora's awareness. She remained with her back to him even when he opened the door and let a beacon of lamplight sweep across the floor and embrace mother and child.

"Good evening, Father," he said, stepping into the hallway and helping the almoner with his rain-soaked cape. In the light Leander's own face bore the power of a father's grief. The raw spring air washed across the vestibule from the entryway. "Please come this way. They're in the parlor."

"I'm truly sorry," Pandora said, her whisper cut with hysteria as she crossed toward them from the parlor. "You cannot possibly come in right now. Francesca has been crying so long I thought I'd go mad but now thank heaven she's just slipped off to sleep. I am sorry but I must insist you postpone your visit until tomorrow." She smiled vacantly, her hands fluttered erratically as if she were some bird directing the enemy from her nesting place.

"It's all right, my child, Francesca is in the arms of the Lord now. She will cry no more."

"No!" Pandora stomped her foot. "It's not all right. I told you she's just gone to sleep. She has no need of a priest. She only needs her mother. She only needs my arms around her, not the Lord's. Now get out, damn you!" She smacked the priest soundly across the face. Leander grabbed her around from behind. Her feet left the ground. She went rigid. Inside she felt a growl begin from deep, deep down. "No, no, you can't waken her! You can't touch her!" She tried to release herself, but Leander held her even tighter against his body. "I'm a doctor, I'll take care of her. She'll be all right."

Leander let her down and held her more gently. "No she won't, my darling. Our daughter is gone. It makes no sense but it is nonetheless true. She is beyond even your loving care."

"Oh, Leander, please, please, don't let it be true our baby is gone." Pandora wailed and collapsed to the floor.

CHAPTER FIFTEEN

"All right, Pandora." Mademoiselle said, throwing open the drapes and allowing the sun into the darkened bedroom. Pandora closed her eyes in shock against the brightness. "You listen to me now. I want you out of this bed at once and I'll have no rebuttal."

"Leave me alone, Mademoiselle. Go away!" Pandora said, watching Mademoiselle take undergarments and petticoats from her cupboard and arrange them on the chair.

"I have left you alone for two weeks. I have watched you starve yourself, drive your grieving husband away, pray to God for death and curse Him for the life He took. But I have come to the end of it. You are not the first mother to lose a child nor will you be the last."

"I know that perfectly well!" Pandora sat up abruptly. "But I don't understand what happened. In the morning all was well; then so quickly, so without warning, she was gone. What horrid thing could have struck her? I must know what curse stole my baby from me."

Mademoiselle took Pandora's chin and turned her resistant head toward her. "They are little frail creatures. Life is stern and harsh. They get sick and they die. It happened to you and it happened to me. The mothers go on. Now get these clothes on. We're going to church. It is mid-Lent and the first decent day we've had this awful spring." Tears fell from Mademoiselle's cheeks despite her preoccupied fuss at arranging and gathering Pandora's outfit.

Pandora had not considered how much the loss of Francesca affected the old woman. She had not thought about how much pain and suffering the death had caused anyone other than herself. But as she watched her old nanny stoically fight to keep her composure, Pandora realized that Mademoiselle was a far grander woman than she had thought even before this last test of strength. "You are right, Mademoiselle. It is a beautiful day. Let us go to church."

***

The mammoth bells of Notre Dame summoned the crowds to prayer. It was a truly glorious day, the sky was a cloudless azure, the air a welcome heraldry to spring. The atmosphere was full of gaiety and festiveness in the midst of these somber days of Lent. Pandora could not help but attract the mood and despite her somewhat weakened legs and deep-seeded sadness, her despair began to soften. She removed her bonnet and turned her face upward to the sun, letting its warmth seep deeply into her exhausted body. Leander held her arm gently, guiding her along.

Mademoiselle was in charge. She had succeeded in drawing Pandora out and God, as she reminded them several times along their route had, aided her with this fine weather. The celebrations were well underway. Each boulevard had become another world of human bodies bearing masks that looked like animal creatures escaped from a Roman myth. Harlequins of all sizes and shapes danced the chahut in little groups that formed at random. The usual buskers and souvenir sellers were barking their goods to the uncostumed legions who were wending their way to their church, or, as were Mademoiselle, Pandora and Leander, they were heading to Notre Dame. On this mid-Lent Sunday, the sobriety of the season was lifted and for Pandora, for the moment anyway, her grief was abated.

"We'll climb to the top of the tower," Mademoiselle said. "The view has no equal and it will lift our spirits to see why God himself preserved this land on which to build his last and greatest cathedral." Mademoiselle's devout faith had not diminished an iota over the years. Pandora marveled at it more than ever before. She felt a little small in comparison, having cursed God so vehemently after Francesca's death. And now that she understood Mademoiselle had suffered the same tragedy, that Francesca's loss was no less felt, she found herself beginning to fight against the pain and self-pity she had been nurturing these past weeks. She would now try to follow the example of Mademoiselle.

"Come, come, my dears," Peliciàn took them both by their hands and pulled them along. "Twenty centimes will soften the heart of the custodian and we'll see the giant clappers that make this lovely ringing." When they arrived at the open plaza in front of the cathedral, Mademoiselle spread her arms wide as if to embrace the entire facade. The sun reflected off the great circular rose window above the central doorway and the power of the intoning bells could be felt in the bottom of one's stomach. "I have often wondered," Peliciàn said, turning to Leander and Pandora, "why the Holy Father in His profound wisdom has not seen fit to move the entire Vatican here. If you ask me, it would be an infinitely better place for the center of our faith."

"I am sure the Italians would argue that with some rigor, Mademoiselle," Leander said, putting his arms around both women's shoulders and looking up at the magnificent edifice.

"They can argue all they want, but that won't make them right. Now let us go inside and give thanks for our blessings. Then we will throw these coins in the reliquy fountain and ask our Lord for a good year to come and to care for our little Francesca:" Her eyes lowered but she did not allow the cloud to dim her spirit long. "Here are your coins." She drew six shiny coins from her pocket and handed Leander and Pandora three each.

Pandora had become distracted by the distinctly foreign call of three wayfarers who were marking a chalk circle on the ground some distance from them. They had taken her attention because they reminded her of the types she had known as a young girl. These were fellows who breezed about all the great cities of Europe. Some places called them tramps and treated them with derision or ridicule, but Paris had always allowed them at least an uneasy welcome. They had slept under the bridges along with the other dispossessed, and in her youth she had listened to their strange broken language and imagined the places of which they spoke. Pandora had planned to let Francesca know all kinds of people including these drifting souls whose free spirits and carefree ways had made such a lasting imprint on her.

"Come along, Pandora," Leander said.

"One moment. I want to watch this trio." One of the men was dressing up as an elephant. He was stuffing his greyish costume with the last bit of paper so that his legs and arms were now quite fat and cumbersome, causing his movements to be lumbering and heavy-looking. He had two large cabbage ears attached to either side of his cap, and a yellow squash swooped out from his own nose and was mounted in such an ingenious fashion that it hung below the fellow's chin and swung like a trunk when he moved. The other two were dressed as harlequins, one with blue diamonds, the other with red. Their satin patches were worn and dull, but their enthusiasm was sharp and energetic. The one with the red was attempting to gather a crowd while the other turned cart-wheels about the periphery of the circle. When a reasonable group had assembled, Pandora among them, the fellow in blue leapt upon the back of the elephant man. This prompted a rocking and swaying from the paper pachyderm and many overly active expressions of terror and trembling from his clinging rider. The ring-master snapped a whip from out of his sleeve. The elephant lifted his arms up and while he stepped right and left in rhythm with the crackling whip he pawed the air. Then the elephant man began to lumber around the edge of the circle, swinging his vegetable trunk and lifting his head up and down, while the rider climbed unsteadily to his shoulders. The crowd applauded once the blue harlequin was atop the beast's shoulders and threw a shower of centimes. The ringmaster spurred the team for more speed with his whip.

Pandora looked around the crowd of people. There were some dressed in costly finery as well as some threadbare, but they all wore expressions of happiness and pleasure at this simple amusement. Paris was such a perfect city to see such sights. Leander flipped two coins which had landed on his hat brim into the circle, then he handed Pandora some of her own to toss.

Just then the elephant man stood up with a jerk. His body was so rigid, the rider tumbled with a hard thump to the ground. The crowd roared its merry approval and applauded vigorously. But Pandora was startled by the nature of the paroxysm. Previously the elephant man had moved with a graceful imitation. It was odd for him to suddenly abandon it for such awkwardness. She stepped a little closer to the circle when the man thrashed in another spasm of movement. He spun around on one leg. His body began to twitch and convulse. He turned toward the crowd and made soundless cries with his mouth. Pandora stood fixed, something looked too familiar to her.

The crowd began to disperse, the now macabre dance losing its appeal. "Pandora?" Leander said, taking hold of her elbow.

"One moment," she said, putting her hand up to keep him away. Just then the man caved in at the knee and went to the ground. As soon as he felt the earth he began to claw viciously at his stomach. It was as if he were trying to retrieve something. His squash nose split against the ground when at last the poor man fell face forward. Pandora rushed to him and placed his head on his lap. She removed the remainder of the play nose and began to wipe the dark blood that seeped from his broken nose. His color was cyanotic blue, his eyes were blank and rolled back, and his head was a solid weight in the well of her lap. He'd soiled himself. He was dead.

Pandora watched the blood spread onto her floral skirt. Something, a glimmer of recognition began to form in her mind the black blood, the unexpected convulsions, the blue skin so fast out of nowhere. She had seen these same things when her little Francesca had gone. Everything the same, and so fast without warning.

"Cholera moribus, Asiatic cholera," she muttered. "Step aside, move away, step aside. What has happened here?" Pandora squinted into the sun. "This man is dead," she said, to the voice whose silhouette was all she could make out.

"Pandora," Leander said behind her, "get up. There is blood soaking your clothing."

"This man is dead," Pandora heard the other man say, and she saw now he was a member of the National Guard. "Get coverings and remove him. Madame, you are getting quite soiled, you'd better get up."

Pandora's mind was far away. She was seeing Francesca again, the sudden erratic movements she made, the blue tinge that colored her once robust little face, and the black blood. It hadn't occurred to her then that this could have been the deadly cholera. How did it invade their home, how had it gotten to Paris? Two guards hoisted the dead clown from Pandora's lap.

"You'd better get some fresh clothing, Madame. You're quite a sight." The first guardsman assisted her to her feet.

"Where are the two others?" she asked, looking around for the red and blue harlequin.

"What two others?" the guard asked, startled by the sharp tone she used.

Then she saw them standing at the edge of the circle. She rushed to them, questions and fears propelling her."Where have you come from?" she asked.

"We came on the barge down the river this morning."

"I asked where did you come from, not how did you come." The two men started to turn away but Pandora grabbed the one in red by the arm and held on hard. "Where have you come from?"

"Excuse me, Madame, but may I ask if you have some connection with these fellows," the tall, long-faced guardsman said, rocking slightly back on his heels. Pandora sensed he did not approve of her aggressiveness. "Tell me," he said to the red harlequin, stepping in front of Pandora, "was this fellow a kin to you?"

"No, just a comrade. We came together to entertain. You know how it is with us. We meet somewhere, the hop harvest or something, and then we link up and travel to the next job. Why, I don't even know his Christian name, Captain. I call him Russian George because he's from Riga."

"Riga!" Pandora shouted, surprising everyone nearby. She looked at the covered corpse, a young priest was serving the last rites. She remembered everything now: the articles in the papers about the cholera, and Riga, where it had started. She remembered the assurances proclaimed that all those coming from the East would be held at the borders to secure our nation's very life. France was prepared. France was safe. The populace must not fear. "Damn, damn!" she cursed. "Tell me, Captain, where will the body be taken?"

"Well, Madame, unless the gentlemen claim him, he will go to the morgue like all the rest who have no one to bury them."

CHAPTER SIXTEEN

Pandora drew up her feet anticipating the sudden resurgence of heat in the copper tub each time Mademoiselle poured the hot water from her bucket into the rising tide of her bath. When all the warmth had evened and the scented bubbles swarmed playfully on the surface, Pandora slid down and rested her head on the cured rim of the tub. She looked over at the cast-off clothes lying in a discarded heap on the chair.

"That's good, child," Peliciàn said, "you have a long soak."

Pandora closed her eyes and listened to the comforting bustle of Mademoiselle's movements about the room. She imagined her laying out the towel and draping her dressing gown over the heated rack.

"I'll put your black satin hair ribbons on your dressing table—they've been pressed."

"Thank you, Madamoiselle," Pandora said, keeping her eyes closed. She heard the door gently close and felt the momentary cool breeze of Mademoiselle's exit.

The vapors from her bubble bath drifted into her nostrils but no matter how pleasant and soothing they were, the smell from her soiled clothes and the dead man's stench remained deeply entrenched in her senses. It seemed the more she tried to wash or will it away, the more pervasively it lingered. What was it that would not be banished? That even her peaceful bath could not quell?

She felt like she was in the middle of some giant puzzle with the pieces swirling about her. She did not know how they fit, but the odor, the noisome odor was absolutely key. She took her wash-cloth and began to wash her face. She remembered now where she had experienced that same smell. It was in Mauritius, when she had been in the wards and cholera had struck. Her uniform had retained the exact malodorous scent that now clung to her bloodstained dress. She shuddered. Francesca had that awful smell, she too had the same cyonosis as the elephant man. Could it be that the cholera had invaded Paris? Why had there been no reports? Perhaps because it wasn't cholera. After all, Francesca's death could have been the result of intero-mesenteric fever. And the elephant man, given the way these vagabonds lived, could have been poisoned, or he too could have suffered the fever. Was she just a mother grabbing at straws? No, deep inside her she sensed she was on to the truth, horrible as it was. But there was only one way to be sure. She had to get the body. An autopsy had to be performed. It was a simple matter, cut him open, see the degree of inflammation in the intestinal mucous and if the muscular rigidity was a pathognomic sign. She slapped the water at the simplicity of it all. Why hadn't she thought of this right off?

"My God!" she said. "The man came from Riga! That's where the epidemic had been born. But how did he get through the border? What did the red harlequin mean when he said they picked him up at the hop harvest? When was that? Had it been days or weeks before today?"

The questions came in a flurry. No one was going to go near that body. An autopsy on an unclaimed tramp? Why? Why would his death set off a medical alert? And France had secured its borders on the East to prevent any threat of cholera.

"Preposterous!" she cursed. There was no security against the cholera! She had to find the answers herself. It was, after all, her duty to report what she believed to be an impending disaster. The question was how would she do this.

Suddenly she started to laugh. "Dr. James Barry, of course!" But her exuberance quickly turned to ridicule. "I'm Dr. James Barry, the English surgeon," she mocked. "I just happened to be in the neighborhood and thought I'd like to do an autopsy this evening. Do you have anyone available? Oh, thank you. I see a gentleman over in that corner, he'll do just fine."

Her laughter made her feel good despite its source. It had been a long time.

"Leander is right," she mused. "When I get wound up I'm quite the ludicrous one. Maybe I could send him as Dr. Barry's emissary. He can certainly be convincing and with a few flashy medical terms— Calm down, Pandora. First I'd have to convince him. Then he'd have to convince an attendant to take one of his superiors away from Sunday dinner just to dig into the gut of some useless fellow all on the directive of a foreigner." An Englishman at that. No, the whole thing was growing more and more absurd. She would have to try to put her faith in God and the keenness of her colleagues.

Then again maybe she was wrong about all this and it really was just a need to find an answer for Francesca's death. But thinking this way had given her some relief from the unrelenting blackness that had engulfed her since her baby died. She slid deeper into the warm water again.

Soon they would return to England and the closeness of family. They would see her through, and this time it would be more complete as Mademoiselle Peliciàn would be there also. Pandora knew now that despite Mademoiselle's dogmatic nationalism and her disdain for a Protestant nation, she would not abandon the family after the last events. Pandora needed her more than ever and Mademoiselle knew it. So in spite of her bias and after a probable fuss only for prides sake, love and devotion would get Mademoiselle Peleciàn to England.

A chill ran across her shoulders. England meant retelling the whole horrible story again. She sank back into that frigid blackness that was never far away. She saw the candles burning—the awful, dim, flickering light, which cast a giant shadow of the cradle on the wall where she had stood vigil. She saw the white lace christening bonnet tied in a bow under her baby's waxen face. So different had it been when she and Leander had first tied the pink ribbon under their rosy newborn's chin.

The water in her tub had not grown cold but Pandora began to shiver. She was trapped, unable to rise from the deep well of her reverie. She took flight in the wings of her dream bird. Flying high above the city, her eye possessed that startling clarity where everything came in her view. She could see at once all of the bridges and boulevards that stretched and wove through the city. She soared and caught the currents of gentle air, then she dove down toward the earth. All along the boulevards and bridges streams of darkly clad, hooded figures were tramping along in a steady lumbering march. As Pandora flew closer she saw that each pair of figures carried a small coffin between them. The procession swelled like an overburdened river as column met column at each corner and intersection. Cries of grief and despair ricocheted off the stone facades and tearing a hole into the silent sky. The canyons of the city reverberated with their echo, its steady lockstep tread of thousands of feet heading toward the Pont St. Michel. All the children of Paris were dead.

Crossing the Pont St. Michel, the bereaved arrived in front of the great edifice Notre Dame. In front was a huge pit filled with quicklime. The gaping scar seared the earth and beckoned the throngs as they arrived. Couple by couple, they came as if in some hypnotic state and as they reached the edge of the pit they threw the contents of their coffins into the waiting abyss. Around the mass grave were rag-fettered creatures barking orders and pointing toward the hole with their fleshless hands. When mothers fell prostrate, clawing the ground in unhindered grief, these creatures shrieked and parodied them with lewd imitation.

"I've got to get to that body!" Pandora leapt up. Forgetting where she was she slid back into the tub and sent a cascade of foamy water onto the floor. "MADEMOISELLE! Come quickly!" she called, grabbing her robe. Just as she reached the door Mademoiselle was coming through with a load of fresh laundry. The wet floor and her imbalanced burden sent her skating. Pandora grabbed her in a bear hug just before the woman lost her balance entirely. "Mademoiselle? I need clothes!"

"Yes, yes, I know. What is it you think I'm carrying here? Grapefruits?"

"No, not these clothes—I need men's clothes!"

"Child, what are you saying?" Peliciàn said dropping her bundle and grabbing Pandora's shoulders. "What happened to you? Has your mind broken? I thought you had finally come out of yourself, and now this foolish request. Tell me why? What has happened?"

"Don't ask questions. Just follow my instructions. I have no time to explain things now."

"Leander!" Mademoiselle called out, but Pandora's earlier cry had already brought him to the door. "Pandora is asking for men's clothing. She's gone off. Lord help us, what has happened to her?"

"Please!" Pandora shouted. "Stop and listen to me, I have not gone off. I know exactly what I am saying, but there isn't time for a lengthy explanation or debate. Mademoiselle, even though we have always honored each others privilege to keep our past our own, I now need to reveal something of mine to you. Please try to accept it as fact without question." Pandora led Mademoiselle to a chair and gave Leander a reassuring look in response to his doubtful one.

"Mademoiselle, I am going to tell you something quite shocking, and I expect you will think a little less of me when I am finished. But I need you to hold judgement until I can further explain and until after I have completed a task."

Mademoiselle Peliciàn sat up rather straight in the chair and jutted her chin forward the way Pandora had so often seen her do when bracing for bad news.

"I am a doctor and surgeon!"

Mademoiselle's eyes gleamed with total incredulity. "I do not understand, child. Doctor? How is this possible?"

"Pure and simple, I went to medical school and passed the necessary requirements to become a medical doctor. Of course I could only achieve this by masquerading as a man. So until I returned to my home in England, I was living as a doctor and a man."

"In the name of the kingdom of heaven!" Mademoiselle exclaimed, looking upward, then to Leander for confirmation that Pandora had truly gone mad.

"What Pandora says is the truth," Leander said, taking hold of the old woman's plaintive hands. "But I don't understand why you are revealing all of this now and with such suddenness."

"Leander, when I was stationed in South Africa I was sent to Mauritius to treat the Asiatic cholera, which had broken out there. Today, while in my bath I realized that something about that elephant man's death and our daughter's were similar. It bothered me so because I knew I'd seen these exact signs somewhere before. Well, it came to me. I had seen this in Mauritius. It was the cholera that I'd seen before, and now I've seen it again."

"Cholera! Mon Dieu!" Peliciàn wailed.

"Pandora," Leander said, "Don't you see what you're doing? You're just trying to understand and control something that you cannot. Why our child was taken from us we cannot answer and even if we could we can't change it. So why are you grasping at such a thin preposterous idea?"

"You're right that I am looking for an understanding, Leander. But it's not out of my grief over Francesca. I saw something that may be far more ominous than two deaths. If I am right in my assumption, there will be many more. I can do something about it, or at least I can try."

"What in heaven's name can you do?" Leander shouted.

"I can autopsy that performer—see if others in the morgue have gone similarly—and, if I'm correct, I'll make someone listen."

"This is just insane, Pandora. Who's going to listen to you?"

"No one will listen to me. But they will listen to Dr. James Barry."

"I forbid it. I absolutely forbid it!"

"Leander, please. I have a plan. Please grant me this wish. I must resurrect James Barry for just one more day."

CHAPTER SEVENTEEN

As a weak setting sun did its best to dry the puddle-strewn streets, the mismatched pair walked full of brisk intention toward their mission. Pandora could not help but notice the strange backward looks they received each time they passed another pedestrian. She had forgotten what it was like to masquerade—the quizzical stares of people upon first sight of someone such as she. Nonetheless she had never been gawked at like this before. She tried to look at it from an outsiders point of view, to see what it was that caused such an extreme reaction. The picture was immediately clear. Here came two rather wild looking creatures, one grand-sized woman marching with charged step, apron tails flapping, bonnet barely keeping her wild mane of hair in control, the other a small sized, overdressed Jack Sprat, who seemed to have borrowed his clothes from a man twice his size.

Just then she stepped on the cuff of her trouser and once again had to stop to readjust Leander's foreshortened braces, which despairingly tried to hold up her high-wasted pants. Of course they stared, she thought, finishing her adjustments. Who wouldn't? Poor Mademoiselle had tried vainly to tailor a passable suit from Leander's, but time and Pandora's impatience had been against her. So now here they were, muddling along with Pandora's appearance very much the cliche stage eccentric. It was all she could do to keep up with Mademoiselle's bold strides and not lose sight of their goal.

As they crossed the Boulevard St. Germaine, Pandora blocked out the scenario for her star player, peppering her instructions with directorial interpretation, while she watched her leading lady for signs of understanding. But Mademoiselle gave no indication that she was paying the least attention and kept marching onward like a statue that had just found legs. Quickly they made their way against the flow of pedestrians, across the Pont St. Michel until they reached the apogee of the bridge where they saw their destination, the Paris Morgue.

Just then an attendant in apron and shirt-sleeves came through the door. With his chicken sized arms he began to wrestle with a bottom-weighted sign. After much struggle he finally managed to rotate it so that it now read "CLOSED." Pandora drew a short, startled breath.

"Please, Monsieur, please!" Mademoiselle screamed suddenly and launched herself forward to the incline of the bridge. "My boy! My boy! I must see my boy!" she shrieked, hurtling headlong down the steep S-shaped walk which led to the morgues entrance. "Give him back to me, I say! He's mine, not yours!" she bore down hard on the frightened keeper, whose baby-thin blonde hair stood up on his head. Quickly, he opened the door and jumped aside with an ungainly demi-pirouette, having obviously learned long ago to avoid confrontation with an inconsolable mother. His thin frame fluttered prissily as Mademoiselle barged through the door. Pandora, close at her heels, nodded to the high-strung young man in a stern, professional manner before he could collect himself and make inquiry.

The public area of the morgue was empty, the last viewers having already left. Pandora's eyes adjusted to the suffused light filtering through the tinted skylight. She surveyed the establishment and was impressed by its order. The room was arranged for optimum viewing with one long glass partition, behind which the "residents" lay on marble tables, wetted down, naked, and still. Their clothes were hanging above their heads from a long pole, which ran the full length of the chamber.

"Edelweiss, my boy! What have they done to you? Blessed Jesus! What has happened?" Peliciàn screamed and ran to the viewing glass, slapping it so hard that it prompted a whimsy in Pandora whereupon she saw all the naked forms on the other side suddenly leave their frozen sleep and sit upright in shocked unison. "Justice, I demand j-u-u-u-stice!" Peliciàn bellowed, wringing her hands.

Then she turned with thunderous menace on the flighty caretaker who had literally tiptoed in and now slunk along the wall, trying to escape to his office. Like a bee-stung bull, Mademoiselle charged, forcing him to buckle at the knees and draw in his cheeks. He swallowed with difficulty as if he were trying to bring down a whole apple. Pandora, seeing that Mademoiselle had taken perfect measure of the boy's character and was in complete control of the situation, watched in the background. "Poisoned!" Peliciàn said, seizing the boy by the waistcoat.

"Poisoned! He's been poisoned!" she cried. Real tears soaked her cheeks as she roughed the keeper side to side. "I demand that an autopsy be performed immediately!"

The shrinking fellow was now reduced to a shivering mass inside his sweat-soaked clothes.

"I am not moving from this damnable hole until I know the cause of my baby boy's death!" Pandora's cue was set, and she came forward, all business, for the final fix.

"Madame, Madame, unhand this poor fellow," she said, holding the hand which ensnared the poor attendant's crimson wrist. "I am sure this lad is more than willing to assist us, Madame." Pandora threw a sympathetic look at the fellow.

"Release him?" Peliciàn asked, holding fast. "I'll turn him loose after I tear him limb-from-limb. They've killed my boy, and if I must go to the guillotine, so be it! But I am taking this one with me! I will even the score no matter the consequence!" She lifted the captured arm to full height. The poor, fey lad, having taken all he could, was about to break down.

"Help me, please!" he implored, his voice a swooning contralto.

Pandora stepped between them and slapped Peliciàn soundly across the face.

"Calm yourself, Madame," Pandora said. "I have told you I would reach the bottom of this, but we cannot have you behaving in such a shocking fashion. Look how you have terrorized this poor fellow. Why, you've nearly driven him to a paroxysm!" She lay her hand on the blond youth's shoulder and took Peliciàn's elbow, gently guiding them toward the door to the slabs. "Madame, be with your son, take his cold hand in yours." Uninhibitedly, Pandora drew back the door to where the bodies lay.

"Edelweiss! Edelweiss!" Mademoiselle blubbered, rushing down the row of wet stiffs until she reached the next to last slab, where the elephant man's remains were laid out. His costume and the remnants of his mask hung dutifully above.

"I really thought she was going to kill me," the attendant stammered, his energy divided between grace toward his savior and wary surveillance of his foe. "Please, sir! I am Mr. Bonald. How can I ever thank you? You have surely saved my life."

"I think that you overstate the case, Mr. Bonald," Pandora demurred. "She is merely a mother distraught in the extreme. Allow me to introduce myself. I am Dr. James Barry, staff surgeon, British Military Corps. I am here in Paris to see to some family business. This poor bereaved woman has been in the service of my family since I was a child. Word reached our residence this afternoon that her son—her last remaining flesh and blood, I might add—had come to an untimely, perhaps suspicious end. I assured the dear lady that I would accompany her to the morgue, examine the body, and get to the bottom of the matter. So if you'd be kind enough to furnish me with proper space and implements, I'd like to get right down to it and put her tortured mind at ease." As Pandora completed these remarks, she offered her hand as a sign of agreement. Inside it she held a large gold coin which she pressed firmly into the befuddled fellow's clammy palm.

***

It had taken one whispered word cupped to the ear of Dr. Broussais, Paris's premier anatomist, to cause a brittle crack from his china plate as he intemperately thrust down his napkin ring. His dining room became uncomfortably hushed. The swells around the table froze in an indecision of etiquette while their host sat stock still at the head of the table, staring back into the face of Bonald, his assistant. Without so much as a bow, he extended apologies to his guests and brusquely took his leave, followed closely by the overwrought Bonald.

Out into the night they sped, the grand doctor, without benefit of a topcoat, against the stiff evening wind, followed by his attendant. The latter, having been so terrorized by Dr. Barry's message, had cared not a wit for propriety when he'd hammered on his supervisor's door.

Finishing the final touches on the corpse for presentation, Pandora was busy exposing a section of the elephant-man's leg when she heard noisy entry from the outer room. She replaced her pins and looked up just in time to see the imposing and elegant figure of Dr. Francoise Broussais as he entered the dissection room, a freshly lit black cigar making a fog of blue smoke around his leonine head. Knowing that delay would only serve to raise uncomfortable questions, she plunged straight away into her exposition.

"I am Dr. James Barry, staff surgeon, British Military Corps. I am sorry to have disturbed you, Dr. Broussais, but, as you will soon see, there was no choice." The dead Russian lay center stage, split open to expose his intimate secrets to the knowing eye.

"I would like you to observe, please, the varying degrees of redness in the intestinal mucosa". Pandora spread apart the innards with her instruments and turned the entrails about to make her point acutely visible. "See how clearly delineated the differences are between sympathetic and idiopathic lesions." Silently, the two odd colleagues stood bathed in the saturnine gaslight, reading the entrails of the corpse.

"It was this irritation that adversely affected the spinal column and produced the concomitant muscular cramps and convulsions. These convulsions then inhibited the contractions of the heart's ventricles, causing the subject to experience the inescapable, pathological effect of circulatory failure." Pandora went to the feet of her subject and pulled back a flap of skin to expose another venue of the human plumbing. "Look, doctor, at the stagnation in the veins and arteries of the legs—the intense blue coloration of the epiderm, a direct and obvious consequence of the dimunation of the aforementioned contractions of the heart's ventricles."

Dr. Broussais repeated Pandora's movements as she returned to the main cavity. The two stood, heads bent low, on either side of the table. As Pandora began to probe the core of the body, she slipped open the spinal sheath with a sure move of her scalpel. "Blood. There it is. That's the clincher. Can you see it?" She looked at Broussais's expressionless face.

"There are three more bodies out there," she said. "And I'll bet my life that they have the identical traces.

She waited, but there was still no change from Dr. Broussais. "This is cholera. Cholera Moribus, I have no doubt."

Dr. Broussais stood there, his jaws locked, hands clenched behind his back. She wondered whether he would allow himself to see it. Or would he be blinded by egoism and fear.

"Your French is native, doctor. I am surprised." The anatomist spoke with the studied approach of a seasoned physician.

"I spent formative years here," Pandora replied.

A little uneasy about where this line of inquiry was leading, she stood still while Dr. Broussais scrutinized her more closely. She could only surrender to his inspection. And put herself at ease by focusing her attention on Bonald, who had remained in the background. Grim resolve seemed to have eroded his boyishness. Undoubtedly, he still worried about the wisdom of his decision to comply with Pandora's demand and fetch his superior away from dinner. Pandora attempted to reassure him with a gentle smile.

"Dr. Barry?" Dr. Broussais began, bringing her back to his scrutiny. "You say there are three more out there in wait, who will show exactly the same etiology as this one." He picked up an ivory-handled probe and methodically retraced Pandora's steps through the beleaguered body of the elephant man.

"Yes, sir, I do," Pandora affirmed, her confidence beginning to return. "Two are young men, the other is an ancient woman. All of them, I would guess from their wardrobes, were rag-pickers."

"Doctor, I realize that the hour is unfavorable, but may I impose upon you—?" Dr. Broussais halted, motioning for Bonald to come closer.

"What is it?" Pandora felt a kind of apprehension building.

"Would you be willing to perform the necessary autopsies on the others with me?" Underneath the calmness of his voice, Pandora detected the edge of urgency. Broussais turned to Bonald. "Do you know which they are?"

"Yes, sir!" Bonald nearly saluted. His total relief so focused on self-interest he could not perceive the graver danger that was about to be confirmed.

"Go and prepare them! The women first," Broussais ordered. "Then rouse the following people."

Pandora watched Broussais write some names on a piece of

paper. She recognized each in turn. They were the power elite of French medicine. It looked like her gamble might be won, but she feared it would be longer than she'd anticipated before she returned to Leander.

CHAPTER EIGHTEEN

A brisk wind from the east announced its presence, churning up the Seine and turning it black. The old river responded with short, choppy waves, which lapped against the quay with the fretfulness of a disturbed sleeper. The afternoon rain, which had seemed a thing of the past, had returned. Drunk with the wind, it spilled itself in sudden torrential bursts, then blinding sheets, pushed along like a rowdy by the bilious gusts.

One by one the equipages of the men on Broussaiss's list pulled up to the entrance of the morgue. Their kerosene lamps did little to penetrate the inundation, and their black tops resounded with the thumps of the heavy raindrops. Each time a soaked horse stopped in front of the door and the coachmen called their arrival, Bonald would poke out the tip of his umbrella, push it open and lift it over himself and the edge of the carriage so none of the distinguished gentlemen would fall unnecessary victim to the vicissitudes of the elements. Bonald fussed over each of these gentlemen like a mother partridge husbanding stragglers into her nest. As per his instructions he billeted them in the administrative offices where a warm fire and a hasty repast of beer and sandwiches had been readied to soften their dispositions while they assembled.

Upstairs, just above their heads, Pandora and Dr. Broussais worked quickly to complete the last of their preparations on the three remaining corpses.

"Excusez-moi, pardonnez-moi," Bonald said, entering the sanctum-sanctorum. Both Broussais's and Pandora's heads perked up in unison. "Dr. Dupuytren has just arrived. Sir, he is the last. I am informing you as requested, they are all here," he said, executing several short nods as he backed to the door.

As the evening had progressed, Pandora had noticed that this strange bird seemed to be charged by the extraordinary events. The thought passed through her mind that, ironically, this fellow would probably do very well in the most severe crises. Clearly the man's frailties had been strengthened by a peculiar mix of heightened vitality. Even she had to admit that though the prospect for the future was grim, she too was thriving on the extraordinariness of the circumstances.

"Bonald!" Dr. Broussais said, forestalling his aide's departure, clipping the tip of yet another cigar with his surgical scissors. "Give us another five minutes and then send them up."

Pandora noticed the change in tone of her prestigious counterpart. No longer was he addressing the obsequious lad as a master does a miscreant servant. Instead he was speaking to Bonald almost as one for whom he had the utmost regard. This subtle shift to the avuncular was not lost on Bonald either. He shone with its receivership.

***

Dr. Broussais stayed with the closed door, then lit his Havana. With a whirl of smoke, he about-faced, the tip of the cigar glowing red as a hot coal. Pandora regarded with considerable attraction the efficiency and esthetic style of his smoking. He exhaled a perfectly metered stream of blue into the room.

"Dr. Barry," he said, his face for the first time neither aloof nor remote toward her. "I fear your findings are correct. I have called the team downstairs for two distinct and hopefully complimentary purposes. Truly, they are the most formidable ad hoc body of medical men one could assemble. Their expertise is nonpareil in each of their respective specialties. So their first function is pure to confirm or deny our grave conclusion.

"But their second function is political, therefore impure and most difficult. Their influence, status and power must be congealed into one unanimous voice, before we leave this room tonight. If we can achieve this, we may be able to get the jump on our deadly foe and ring the tocsin bell in time to avert a disaster of Homeric proportions."

"But surely, Doctor," Pandora said. "With the facts so clear, there can be no cause for dissension among trained men."

"Ah ha!" Broussais exhorted. "Now I know who, or should I say what, you are."

"What do you mean?" Pandora's throat tightened.

"I kept asking myself, all evening, who is this strange little fellow and why is he here? Why is he doing this with his Sunday evening? It makes no sense. I could see no causal relationship. Now it is all clear, you are an idealist! A rare thing to find in a doctor, rarer still in a military man. But you must never forget my friend, that even in the face of the worst foe, the petty academic rivalries born out of our professions and competition for glory, often, I would dare say almost always, take precedence over the facts and service of the populace."

Broussais began to pace up and down between the tables upon which the three open corpses lay. "Among the men at the top of any profession there are histories, ones which have yielded wounds and scars. Some are deep and some are jagged, but all are painful. They are the result of battles fought on the fields of ideology and belief."

He stood still and drew upon his cigar. "In order that the waters do not become more choppy than they already are, I am asking that you put yourself in my hands. Specifically that you allow me to present our case and its arguments in my own way."

Pandora bowed an immediate assent. After all, given the circumstances, she was in his hands by default, therefore she had no choice but to acquiesce. She did not even bristle at his putting her in the secondary role. She had liked him from the first—his measured speech, his thoughtful ear and even the rich pleasure he derived from his cigar. These simple traits reassured her of his basic goodness. Before he had spoken of scars she had already traced his. She had no doubt that he was a doctor who had forged his reputation in the clinical laboratory, not in the salons where so many others in a cosmopolitan society can find a criterion for advancement. She suspected that he was much more the idealist than she.

"Whatever you think best, doctor. I do have one reservation though, but I think it can be cleared up quickly if you'll permit a question."

"By all means!" Broussais replied.

"Was your service in the army or navy, sir?" she asked.

"Navy." He knitted his brows.

"Well, then..." Pandora smiled lightly. "That clears it up. Since this part of the building sits over the water it's only appropriate that the army man be junior to the navy."

The fraternal joke was cut short by the noisy entry of the minion, led by Bonald. Pandora eased inconspicuously from center stage to a ringside position in the corner and observed the entrants. Each one declared his prominence either by the distinguished turn of his mustache, the superb cut and fit of waist of his frock coat or the exaggerated carriage of his head and chest. As they exchanged terse greetings with Dr. Broussais, Pandora tried to match names with notability. She smoothed the lapels of her ill-fitting coat to gain a better line just in case she should soon be introduced. But as the gentlemen became aware of the three cadavers on the table and took note of their condition, Pandora's presence faded further into the corner. While she expected this she did fret a bit at the impression she might make on this August gathering. She became increasingly aware of her appearance and again made an effort to adjust her ill-fitting garments.

Just then she noticed among them a tall figure who was standing aloof from the others. He was wearing a spectacular military uniform that was bedecked with abundance of medals. His physique was slender. He stood rigidly erect with his hand resting on the hilt of his sword in such a natural way that one seemed an extension of the other. He had silvery hair, but his mustache was of a hue seen only in portraiture. This gentleman alone had noticed Pandora in her unobtrusive position and when she caught his eye, he acknowledged her with a slight bow. Her savvy told her he had something to do with the king. What was he doing here?

"Gentlemen," Broussais started. "Let me begin by begging your forgiveness for the unfortunate timing of my summons. But when we have finished our proceedings I believe you will understand the urgency of this gathering."

"Don't play the professor with us," Dupuytren said, removing his coat, and getting closer to one of the cadavers. "You're convinced the cholera has arrived, and you need corroboration.

Broussais, you know how much I hate gamesmanship, so let us get to business without further hesitation."

At once the room turned into a workplace. Off came coats and cravats. Stiff collets were untied from necks and dropped over stool tops. A din of conversation arose as instruments were chosen, and the prodding and snipping began. The sense of prestige that had impressed Pandora when these men arrived now turned to tremendous admiration. Without the least hesitation all of them had jumped right into the fray and, despite Broussais's words to her earlier, it had appeared for the present egos had been put aside.

Pandora remained in the corner, spellbound. Each of these men went about his task with a vitality and focus so intense, she understood why all of them were so esteemed. She had a moment of envy, if only just to participate with them. Just then the tall commander came over and stood close to her, nodding acknowledgment before he returned his focus to the action around the dissecting tables.

"I'll say one thing right now," Dupuytren hollered, lifting his head away from the old woman he was probing. "I don't know yet what killed her, but this old gal had quite a case of pneumonia and, judging from the state of these wind bags, it wasn't her first bout."

"Gentlemen, come here and look at this!" Recamier called from the other side of the pneumoniatic woman. "Observe the swelling of the ilio-caecal valve and the formation of the mesenteric glands." By the brash, rather over-assured manner with which he addressed the others Pandora deduced Racamier was the junior among them.

"I for one reject the idea of cholera," he said, thumping the table with the thin end of his instrument as the others peered into his cadaver. "This old girl is clearly a case of intero-mesenteric fever, not cholera."

"Pompous fool." Pandora muttered under her breath. She couldn't stop her leg from commencing an irritated tap as she itched more and more to get there and show them all how utterly clear her diagnosis had been. The shackle of her promise to Dr. Broussais was not such an easy task for her, especially when she had to listen to such arrogant ignorance as this.

Her restiveness drew the attention of the solider next to her but she was too preoccupied to care at this point. This congress of experts was not approaching the matter properly. How in heavens name could they be missing it? Her envy was turning to smoldering impatience.

"You're looking through the wrong end of the telescope, young man," Broussais's voice rose above the din of sarcasm and sniping that had begun as a result of Recamier's remarks. "What you observe is correct, Joseph, but your extrapolation is completely off. What you are seeing is the result of sanguinary congestion, not fever! This congestion involved the entire digestive tract, which no doubt caused severe muscular cramps. It ultimately affected the spinal column, producing convulsions and finally paralysis of the heart. The demise is rather quick but it is preceded by a terrible suffering. We only see the aftermath, gentleman. Do we want to ignore the clear classification that is indicated here? If we do, I fear we will be seeing a lot more horror."

Pandora saw how tenuous a grip the doctor held on the contentious group. Soon he would lose them to the mire of intellectual combat, and any notion of discovery or alarm would vanish. Immediately fulfilling her prophecy, the group dissolved into chaos, everyone talking at once, each propounding his own self-assured conviction. Pandora stood helplessly by as they fragmented and fractured into so many cantankerous children, one snatching hold of the remark of another in order to condemn or deride his view.

The commander, who had stationed himself half on and half off a high three-legged stool near the wall, swung his leg over to dismount. Then, mantled with a grand presence, he strode into the fray. He took ground between Dr. Broussais and the antagonists without a wasted movement. The effect of his power was imperious. These heretofore petulant men became still, even gazing slightly downward as they shuffled into a semi-circle around the consul. For a few moments the commander did nothing to relieve the tension. On the contrary, it seemed to Pandora, his intention was to let them stew. He moved his eye slowly from party to party in a particular way that intimated a threat, then he broke it off with a smile which displayed a set of teeth as top caliber as his mustache.

"I did not mean to interrupt Messrs.," he said in a voice that made Pandora think of the outdoors. "But may I be permitted a question?"

All the doctors fell over themselves with foolish assents, each trying to be the more gracious. "Everyone has voiced one opinion or another with great zeal and authority, but two of us have yet to be heard from. I myself cannot project a view as I am merely a marshal of the royal service, but I have been observing the gentleman in the corner quite closely. By his impatience I would assume he has an opinion on the matter at hand. I for one am curious as to what it is and who he is."

Pandora felt a blush grow from her feet to the top of her head as all eyes fell directly on her. But before she could make any adjustments Dr. Broussais had taken her arm and brought her into the light.

"Marshal Oudinot, gentlemen," he said. "This is Dr. James Barry, staff surgeon of the British Medical Corps, a longtime friend and colleague of mine and one who has extensive experience with the cholera. Today he paid me an unexpected call as he is in France on some personal matters. Fortuitously, his visit has coincided with the arousal of my suspicions in the cases before us and I presumed on his friendship and impressed him to lend a hand." Pandora was pleased to see that Dr. Broussais was a capable, high-quality liar.

"I see, Dr. Broussais," Marshall Oudinot said, then turned his attention to Pandora. "I am quite sure one as eminent as Dr. Broussais has not exaggerated your worth or expertise one iota and we are grateful for your assistance, Dr. Barry, but since you are here among us, would you now be so kind to break your silence and share with us your views on our present conundrum?"

Pandora's heart beat soundly. Here she was surrounded by medical eminence and the King's own representative. She had no time to worry about her secret or how she might appear to them. She only knew that they were to listen. She had to make certain they got her message. She stepped away from the protection of Dr. Broussais. The strength of her conviction gave her a solid voice.

"Marshal Oudinot, gentlemen," she said, "there is one thing I would like to point out to you immediately. A piece of evidence that perhaps may tip the scales of your inquiry." She started to remove her jacket but thought better of it. "Would you all now open the spinal envelopes of each of your subjects."

A bustle of activity ensued while the medical men including Dr. Broussais proceeded. The thrill of purpose invigorated her. "Dr. Megendie," she said. "Since this falls into your specialty, would you personally examine each one of the spinal canals?" The middle-aged doctor, whose hair was combed forward to conceal his baldness, moved towards the old woman's body. Dr. Recamier and Dr. Dupuytren demurred to their colleague whose tie still remained tight at his throat. "If you find, sir," Pandora's voice now rang full of confidence, "traces of blood in the cord and envelope of each case, would you not agree that we have present nothing other than cholera moribus?"

"Yes, I would, sir." Silence took hold of the room as Dr. Megendie went from corpse to corpse, methodically examining each exposed spinal cord. Then he came to the center of the room and looked directly at Pandora. "Gentlemen," he said. "Our British colleague is absolutely right. I am afraid there is no doubt that the cholera has arrived in Paris."

CHAPTER NINETEEN

In the hubbub of activity pursuant to Dr. Megendie's proclamation, Pandora once again became the outsider, regaining her anonymity amidst the ensuing debate. "Mission accomplished, objective secured," she whispered with both self-satisfaction and relief. Then from the protection of her corner, she stood and watched Marshall Oudinot watching the others. He did not move or react in any outward way, nor did he try to impose himself on any one of the myriad debates now pervading the room. He simply stood as erect as ever and studied and waited.

Suddenly, his role in these proceedings was crystal clear. If in fact the cholera epidemic had arrived in Paris the government would be faced with not only a grievous health hazard, but also a political situation of the highest sensitivity. The Marshall was here to make sure there would be no loose cannons rattling about. Pandora realized her situation had become very precarious indeed and she had not a moment to lose in making her exit and having Dr. Barry disappear from whence he came.

Using the cover of medical closure, she made her way toward the door. She returned a stray instrument to its appropriate case, took a wayward smock from the back of a chair, and delivered it to its rightful hook, which was advantageously located over the wash basin, one brief step from the door. She washed her hands with deliberate care, but watched with feline stealth for her moment. When Oudinot's back was squarely to her, she disappeared in a magicians wink through the exit. With a smoothness of pace she made her way down the shadowy stairwell staying close to the wall. The eerie patches of illumination that flickered onto the steps from the nearly expired wall sconces would guide her footfall. Reaching the bottom, she leaned into the burdensome door and set her sights toward Pont St. Michel.

A gathering of hackney drivers and some of Marshall Oudinot's troops blocked her path. The soldiers were barely visible in the predawn light, but as she entered the courtyard they became alert to egress.

"What say ye, doc, ain't them about done up there?" A gravely voiced driver flagged her as she circumscribed the knot of men whose lot of waiting in attendance knitted them tight together.

"Patience, my man," she said, over her shoulder. "Things are in motion." She kept a casual air but maintained a keen eye on the bridge ahead, evoking as best she could the character of the drained worker out for a bit of fresh air.

A loud burst of laughter broke the quiet and stimulated Pandora to put more distance between herself and them. At the bridge she gradually increased her gait but covered her cross by slipping her hands into her pockets and pausing to gaze aimlessly about the heavens. At the knoll she paused again and looked into the Seine where, a fine mist was riding atop its calmed flow.

Then she turned for one final look at the neo-Greek edifice of the morgue. What she saw froze her. Standing next to one of his guards was the unmistakable figure of Marshal Oudinot. Though light was still elusive Pandora was certain she saw the guardsman pointing in her direction. She did not hesitate any further. At least she'd had foresight and was already in the lead.

As she darted down the bridge and reached the river bank, she turned toward the Pont Neuf. She kept a calm steady pace, knowing that she'd have to conserve some energy for the possibility of a dash. Plus, she needed to gather her thoughts now for a plan.

If she could reach the other side of the Pont Neuf with a substantial lead, then she could sprint to Les Halles where the bustle of the mornings opening would serve as a perfect place to lose her pursuers. She looked back. A group of guards were just gaining the rise. She dug in for more speed.

"Dear God," she said, "please, if I could just reach the Pont Neuf."

She heard the fall of quickening boots on the quay behind her. No looking back. She regulated her breath and sharpened her mind on her route.

"Poise, poise is the key. Panic will defeat me." She ran below the boulevard, the growing light not yet touching her there. Perhaps she'd find a place to conceal herself and let the hunters pass by. The terrain was unsteady. She had to go carefully, but she knew these parts well, and the irony of her present situation did not elude her.

Destiny seemed to be calling her back. Yet again she ran, imperiled and in the dark, from an ardent foe, only it was no longer "L'Homme de la Boite" and she was no longer an orphan child. She was a grown woman, a wife, Leander's wife. She had to return to him. She'd promised. She could not betray that promise. She clung to the sweaty embankment picking her way as daybreak diminished her odds for success. The Pont Neuf was in sight. All she had to do now was scale the embankment. That was easy she knew the tricks, and her size would be an asset. Once she started across the bridge, she could dodge in and out of the activity that would be commencing with the dawn.

"Ya! Yaw! Humph!" she heard the cry as her foot kicked against something that felt like a cabbage. She teetered off balance, flailing her arms to gain control as her whole body hurled forward in flight and then she saw black as she hit the ground. She tried desperately to fill her tired lungs with air.

"You whoreson," she heard above her. She tried to roll over and push herself up, but a weight landed on her neck. She gagged and when her eyes cleared, she saw a giant vagrant looking over her. He had his hand over his ear and blood was running from it into his unruly beard. "I'll smash you like a cockroach!" he howled, lifting a large cobblestone above his wounded head. His three waistcoats spread out like bat wings, enhancing his raging enormity. Pandora struggled to unfix his bare foot from her throat. She tossed her head furiously from side to side to unbalance him.

Several camouflaged clochards rose up from under the rags, sacks and papers into which Pandora had unceremoniously plunged. They cleared away from the impending pummeling without display of excitement or concern, wearily rising and shuffling about as one routinely responds to the cock crow. Suddenly a figure with Medusa-like red hair leaped onto the back of the tramp.

"Coppers! The coppers!" she screamed, attempting to unshackle his mind from murder. Yanking his hair with one free hand, she finally succeeded in drawing his focus from Pandora. But just as fast, the vagrant sent the woman to the ground with the back of his fist. "The Sergot, the bloody head-busters, you damn fool!" she screeched, pointing to the charging guardsmen whose bayonets where at the ready.

The vagrant reckoned the posse, then shot an evil eye on Pandora. "Freaky, squeaky, queer little bastard!" he snarled, hurling the stone into the Seine. Then he grabbed his bundle and followed the fleeing band, which was scurrying like little black beetles disturbed by a sudden intrusion of light, up the embankment.

Pandora rolled over. The pack of hounds was bearing down on her. She forced herself to her feet but a bolt of excruciating pain shot up her right leg and sent her back to the ground. She must have turned her ankle in the fall, but this was no time to think about it. She rose again and made for the lip of the quay. The river was her only hope. If she could not run, let the Seine run for her. She fell to her knees and began to crawl. They were almost upon her. She swung her exhausted body over the edge, resigned to risk it all, when a firm hand landed vice-like on her padded shoulder and clenched her so tightly that she had to squeeze her eyes to stop the tears. Her legs futilely kicked the air as she dangled over the river trying to free herself.

The guard's grip tightened, and he began to pull her upward as other hands reached for her. She quickly grabbed her captor's sleeve and, with every last ounce of strength, she pulled herself up and planted her teeth as hard as possible into this wrist.

"Bastard!" he screamed. But she dug in again until her own jaw felt pain and suddenly she was free, plunging toward the Seine. She went under hard, the cold water filling her uniform. She ripped her jacket off and kicked out of her boots. When she resurfaced she coughed and choked as she fought to get air. Already the fast current had pulled her downstream and toward the middle of the river. She could see her captors in the distance dashing up and down, the one she'd bitten shaking his wounded fist at the black water. She dove under the water again, and with the current speeding her along, she made her way to the opposite bank.

CHAPTER TWENTY

"You've not changed at all. You're still a crazy, ragamuffin child. You could have drowned." Mademoiselle said as she poured the last bit of hot water into the basin where Pandora's feet were planted. Her twisted ankle was a purplish blue and twice its normal size. She was wrapped in flannels and wool and Mademoiselle had brewed a horrible concoction of herbs to warm and cleanse her insides from the hour in the river. She could not seem to get warm. Leander was putting yet another log on the fire in their bedroom fireplace to help speed her thaw.

"Well, my darling," he said, not with a full tone of sympathy. "This was quite an adventure you had. I would say that Dr. Barry has made his last exit from the world in the style of grande finale." Pandora did not comment. She was reviewing the day's events. "What's wrong? Are you still not feeling well?"

"Leander," she said, loosening her wraps, her body coming around. "We came back to Paris, the place of my beginning, to unravel the knot that had started here. I thought as well as you did that I would clearly see who and what I am. With you by my side I thought it would be an easy task. Had our baby lived perhaps everything would have been different."

Leander stiffened.

"Why don't I like the sound of all this? What exactly did you discover, Pandora?" He made himself busy with a smoking log at the fire.

"Well, I found out two things, really, which is why I am speaking to you with such hesitation."

"Pandora, just go on and say everything."

"I'm trying to be clear. Try not be angry right off and make assumptions. Today I realized that I am without a doubt a doctor. It is not just something I learned to do, it's something I've become. For whatever reason, God put it into my blood, even before I discovered it was there. To turn my back on it now would be a sin and a lie of much greater magnitude than my masquerade."

Leander seemed to pale in the amber light of the fire. She got out of her footbath and knelt at his knees, wrapping her arms around his legs. "I also discovered that I love you more than life itself. That all the nobility of being a doctor does not minimize the grandeur of being your wife. I have always remembered what Mr. Barry said so long ago when he was dying. He was right, you know. Our lives are inextricably intertwined, but now what are we to do about it? How do I go on being a doctor and a wife, too? I cannot give up either one."

Suddenly Leander lifted Pandora up and placed her on his lap. He looked at her a long time, his eyes turning warmer and warmer, so that she became so attuned to his silent declaration of love that she began to cry.

"I remember the day you convinced Lord Buchan to sponsor you at Edinburgh. You said something about how one resolves two conflicting facts by the use of a stratagem which satisfies that conflict in its simplest way."

"Occam's Razor?" Pandora said.

"Yes, that was it. You'll just have to do both," he said.

"I don't understand what you mean."

CHAPTER TWENTY-ONE

"Responsibility, Dr. Barry, is the operative word here. You must know that the British military is not some frivolous organization from which one can absent himself without explanation whenever whim or fancy beckons." Pandora dropped her eyes and rotated her cocked hat slowly in her hands, presenting as repentant a figure as she thought effective. "You do know, I presume, that I have been petitioned on your behalf by an extraordinary array of influence? The Earl of Buchan, a personage who cannot be contradicted easily, visited me personally along with Major Miranda to plead on your behalf."

"Major Miranda, a man with whom I had the honor to serve in the Peninsular War, not only spoke with some eloquence and sympathy regarding your position, but has requested you be assigned as staff surgeon in his regiment, the Ninety-Fifth Rifles of the Royal Marines. Naturally, he assured me that he would personally oversee your conduct and take full responsibility. I am reluctant to give way and ignore your actions, but as I stated right off, you seem to be surrounded by a solid sphere of high authority." Pandora smiled a little too self-assuredly, but out of respect covered it with a quick "Yes, sir."

Sir James McGrigor paced back and forth behind his shining wooden desk, puffing vociferously on his pipe. "I am going to sign these documents of transfer, sir, but before I do, I would at the least like some explanation of your mysterious absence." Pandora rose to full attention, filling out her uniform.

"For the record, sir," she said, running her hands through her cropped hair. "Let us say I returned to England to have my hair cut."

EPILOGUE

May 1865

The winds blew against the windows, drying some of the wetness that had gathered on the panes from the violent rains that had gone on since the night before. Leander looked out and watched the clouds buffet across the slate sky above the city. "Perhaps it would be unwise for us to attend the graduation ceremony after all," he said. "I think sitting in the damp chairs on the Common is not such a good idea, your having been somewhat unwell of late."

Pandora laughed, "Not so! You're losing your senses in your old age." She sat in her dressing gown reading, her face quite pale but cheerful despite her bouts of indisposition, which had been aggravated by the extreme and unseasoned heat of this May. "Do you think that I would miss the graduation of Edinburgh Medical School's first woman doctor? If I were on my death bed, I'd be there."

"Pandora," Leander turned and smiled at her. His hair was all white, but his lined face was still handsome and strong. He resembled his father even more than in his youth, but his smile always had his mother's warmth and spark in it. "In point of fact, Elizabeth Anderson is really the second woman doctor to graduate from Edinburgh. It seems to me she is 50 years late."

"Yes, my darling," Pandora said, rising and kissing him lightly on the cheek. "You and I know that, but she doesn't. Now, after all that we've been through, if a little rainy weather is going to kill me, then let it be. Come along, let's dress, I don't want to be late."

Amazingly the rain, which had returned, ceased just as Leander and Pandora's carriage arrived at the Common, where seating had been arranged for the forthcoming ceremony. Captain Johnson, a sturdy soldier, crisp and efficient, opened their carriage door. "Inspector-General Barry, General Miranda," he said, holding the door steady, as the two retired soldiers alighted. Pandora's blue uniform was a perfect fit on her aged but trim and erect figure. Leander, tall and straight, was the picture of military elegance.

As the graduates were receiving their parchments, the sun burst through the grey and dried all the dampness from the air. When Elizabeth Anderson stood to receive her medical degree, the audience, already high in enthusiasm, was greatly warmed, and they provided a rousing applause toward her. Pandora and Leander joined, though in a more subdued way.

"Now, what do you say to this, Inspector Barry?" Captain Johnson leaned closer to her from his chair. "A woman doctor."

"All I can say, young man," Pandora said, "is I thank the good Lord that I am old. After all, who knows what will come next?"

The End

ABOUT THE AUTHORS

Anne Kronenfeld—previously wrote and published *Echos from the Schoolyard* with George Kalinsky (Hawthorne Books). Anne has worked in numerous aspects of the entertainment industry. After a distinguished classical dance career, including performing with New York City Ballet, Anne pursued an acting career. Her film appearances include Woody Allen's *Manhattan, Dancer* (Documentary), and repertory work at the Worklight Theater in New York. Anne has also produced *Staged Work*, cast for stage and television shows, as well as consulted on productions and special events.

Ivan Kronenfeld, Ph.D.—is currently a principal of Koerner Kronenfeld Partners, a conceptual capital company dealing primarily in the entertainment industry: Broadway, Off-Broadway, Book Packaging, TV documentaries, Merchandising and Film Financing. He has more than thirty years experience in experience as an actor, director, producer and writer. Ivan has also worked extensively in academia as both professor and administrator. He previously sold two screenplays.

Made in the USA
Monee, IL
04 November 2026

67382850R10154